To Improve Health and Health Care 2001

Stephen L. Isaacs and
James R. Knickman, Editors
Foreword by Steven A. Schroeder

To Improve Health and Health Care 2001

The Robert Wood Johnson Foundation Anthology

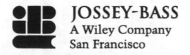

JOSSEY-BASS
A Wiley Company
San Francisco

Jossey-Bass books and products are available through most bookstores. To contact Jossey-Bass directly, call (888) 378-2537, fax to (800) 605-2665, or visit our website at www.josseybass.com.

Substantial discounts on bulk quantities of Jossey-Bass books are available to corporations, professional associations, and other organizations. For details and discount information, contact the special sales department at Jossey-Bass.

Library of Congress Cataloging-in-Publication Data

To improve health and health care 2001 : the Robert Wood Johnson
Foundation anthology / Stephen L. Isaacs and James R. Knickman, editors ;
foreword by Steven A. Schroeder.— 1st ed.
    p. cm. — (Jossey-Bass health care series)
  Includes bibliographical references and index.
  ISBN 0-7879-5276-1 (alk. paper)
    1. Robert Wood Johnson Foundation.   2. Public health—Research
grants—United States.   3. Public health—United States—Endowments.
4. Medicine—Research grants—United States.   I. Isaacs, Stephen L.
II. Knickman, James.   III. Series.
  RA440.87.U6 T6 2001
  362.1'0973—dc21   00-010983

FIRST EDITION
PB Printing   10 9 8 7 6 5 4 3 2 1

—ᴴᴴ— Table of Contents

—ᵚᵚ— Foreword

Now in its fourth year, the *Anthology* series attempts to offer an unvarnished and in-depth analysis of The Robert Wood Johnson Foundation's activities as seen by both insiders and outsiders. Complementing our *Annual Report*, special reports, *Advances*, and Grant Results Reports, the series is one of the ways that we provide an accounting of our programmatic activities to the health field, philanthropy, and the general public. This year's *Anthology* contains ten chapters, the first two of which offer insights from senior staff members into the way the Foundation operates.

In chapter 1, Michael McGinnis, a senior vice-president of the Foundation, and I examine the dramatic shift that took place in 1999 when the Foundation moved from a predominant focus on health care services to one giving equal importance to behavioral and social health. We analyze the reasons for the shift, discuss the major reorganization that accompanied it, and explore the implications for future programming.

Except for a six-year period ending in the early 1990s, Frank Karel has directed The Robert Wood Johnson Foundation's communications unit since its inception in 1973. In chapter 2, he takes a personal and candid look at the Foundation's communications program, tracing its development from the first newspaper accounts announcing the Foundation's creation through its recent use of the Internet. In the bargain, he makes a strong case for strategic communications as an integral part of any foundation's activities.

The next six chapters examine a broad spectrum of Foundation-supported programs.

In chapter 3, Sharon Begley, a senior editor at *Newsweek*, and Ruby Hearn, a senior vice president of the Foundation, chronicle the approaches the Foundation has adopted to improve children's health. Among other things, the authors note that the Foundation has moved from funding demonstration programs designed to spark support from the federal government to supporting large community coalitions.

In chapter 4, Janet Firshein, a journalist specializing in health care, and Lewis Sandy, executive vice president of The Robert Wood Johnson Foundation, take a similarly long perspective. They relate how the Foundation's approach to managed care has changed over the years—from supporting nonprofit group health plans in the 1970s to funding an accrediting agency to develop quality of care standards in the 1980s to encouraging health maintenance organizations to serve chronically ill individuals in the 1990s.

Chapter 5, by Joseph Alper, a journalist who writes about health, and Rosemary Gibson, a senior program officer at the Foundation, examines a series of programs aimed at improving the care of poor older Americans. They find that integrating both the services themselves (acute, chronic, and supportive) and the financing of those services by Medicare and Medicaid is a challenge, and document the ways in which Foundation-funded programs have attempted to foster such integration.

Under the Workers' Compensation Health Initiative, the Foundation funds research into ways to improve the workers' compensation system. In chapter 6, Allard Dembe and Jay Himmelstein, the co-directors of the initiative, summarize the key findings from this research, especially research on ways to integrate the traditional health care system and the workers' compensation system, thus providing what is known as 24-hour coverage. The authors suggest ways in which findings from the initiative can be applied in making workers' compensation more responsive to both injured workers and employers.

In chapter 7, journalist Digby Diehl, describes Sound Partners for Community Health, a partnership with the Benton Foundation in which local public radio stations collaborate with service organizations in their community to provide more and better coverage of health issues. Unlike many programs featured in the *Anthology* series, Sound Partners is a small initiative that is designed not to affect national policy but to increase awareness and improve health in local communities.

Chapters 8 and 9 look back at two areas that the Foundation championed in the 1970s and 1980s.

In chapter 8, Marguerite Holloway, a contributing editor of *Scientific American*, recounts how the Foundation's efforts stimulated and helped shape the development of regional perinatal care networks to identify and care for low-birthweight babies. Although these networks took off in the 1980s, competition among hospitals for neonatal intensive care units and the rise of managed care in the 1990s undermined the idea of regional services.

During the 1970s and 1980s, the Foundation worked to strengthen public health dentistry. In chapter 9, Paul Brodeur reviews the range of programs the Foundation supported to improve the nation's oral health. Although the Foundation did not actively support dentistry in the 1990s, oral health has re-emerged as an area of interest, and new Foundation programs are under development.

This year's *Anthology* concludes with an examination of partnerships among national foundations, complementing a chapter that appeared in last year's *Anthology* on partnerships between The Robert Wood Johnson Foundation and local foundations.

In chapter 10, using Robert Wood Johnson Foundation collaborations as their starting point, Stephen Isaacs and John Rodgers, both from Health Policy Associates, find that, despite rhetoric to the contrary, national foundations do not often enter into collaborations with one another, and that when they do, the partnerships are difficult to maintain. The authors offer suggestions for improving the likelihood of successful partnerships.

As I wrote in the foreword to an earlier *Anthology,* any single volume will provide only a partial view of what The Robert Wood Johnson Foundation does, but over the years a more complete picture will emerge. That picture is now beginning to take shape, and we are beginning to gain insights from the *Anthology* series. In the editors' introduction that follows, Stephen Isaacs and James Knickman offer ten grantmaking insights from the first four volumes. We expect more to emerge in the coming years.

Princeton, New Jersey   Steven A. Schroeder
August 2000   President
The Robert Wood Johnson Foundation

—~— Editors' Introduction

Grantmaking Insights from The Robert Wood Johnson Foundation *Anthology*

Book reviews, letters we've received, and personal comments from readers suggest that the *Anthology* series provides an understanding of The Robert Wood Johnson Foundation in three ways.

- First, by making public the Foundation's decision-making processes and revealing the thinking of key people involved in programs, the series helps demystify the Foundation and the work of its grantees.
- Second, by providing critical, unbiased analyses of the programs the Foundation has supported—many of them written by award-winning journalists—it provides insights into what has worked, what has not, and why.
- Third, by offering a panorama of the Foundation's investments from 1972 to the present, it enables readers to understand the approaches and the strategies that the Foundation has adopted to improve the health and health care of all Americans.

In last year's *Anthology,* we offered some insights based on the first three volumes in the *Anthology* series. In this fourth volume, we expand on that base and identify a number of others. The ten insights on grant making gleaned from The Robert Wood Johnson Foundation *Anthology* follow below:

1. The Importance of Mission and Basic Values

The mission of The Robert Wood Johnson Foundation, "to improve the health and health care of all Americans," shapes the Foundation's culture, guides its investment strategies, and establishes program limits. It is complemented by four core values: pursuit of goals important to the public's health; reliance on data; speaking through grantees; and employing an expert staff.[1] The mission and the core values give the Foundation both a clear identity and a solid base from which to pursue its more specific goals—increasing access to health services, improving chronic care, and combating substance abuse. They also give the Foundation a stability that allows it, through its programs, to advance ideas that might not be popular at any given time, such as increasing the opportunities for minorities to become health professionals, promoting generalist medicine, and combating addiction to tobacco.

2. Staying Ahead of the Curve

Foundations generally want to stay ahead of the curve—to play a leadership role by supporting innovative ideas that will be adopted by others. But how does a foundation staff member—or anybody, for that matter—know where the curve is, much less how to stay ahead of it?

To a great extent, as the *Anthology* series demonstrates, it is through the efforts of a highly professional staff and expert consultants who identify—"sense" might be a better word—areas that are at the point where Foundation support could make a difference. The *Anthology* provides many such examples. During the 1970s and 1980s the Foundation invested in emergency medical services, regional perinatal care networks, and training of nurse practitioners and physician assistants. None of these was in the foreground when the Foundation first took action, but interest in them was stirring, and some health professionals were predicting that they were likely to become important to the health of the American public. As it happens, all three areas developed so rapidly that the contribution of The Robert Wood Johnson Foundation cannot easily be distinguished from the changes made outside of its programs. By supporting early efforts in these fields, however, the Foundation helped propel their development and guide them as they grew.

A more recent example is the Foundation's work on the issue of the harm caused by tobacco. By the 1980s, the evidence was well-established and the tobacco problem was catching attention. Yet no major foundation was directly engaging the issue. In the early 1990s, The Robert Wood Johnson Foundation began to play a role by funding research, policy analysis, anti-smoking coalitions, and a variety of other programs. Although it is difficult to separate the Foundation's role from the changes that took place in society during the 1990s, the

Foundation clearly was ahead of the curve. More recently, the Foundation has turned its attention to addressing unhealthy behaviors and to a new field called "population health," taking advantage of recent data and a sense among many health professionals that these are areas of growing importance.[2]

3. Shaping Public Debate and Perceptions About Difficult-to-Solve Issues

Even a foundation that provides grants of over $400 million a year can expect to have only a limited impact in a trillion-dollar-plus health economy. Many problems, such as drug addiction and the high number of uninsured families, appear all but intractable. Another insight from the first four volumes of the *Anthology* series is that despite an apparent powerlessness to bring about immediate and dramatic changes in society, foundations can keep an idea alive, even though it has not gained wide popular acceptance, and can work to influence the way opinion leaders and the broad public perceive issues.

Take generalist medicine. Although The Robert Wood Johnson Foundation was swimming against the specialist current for many years, its persistent efforts lent stature to the idea that more generalist physicians were needed, and its grants to medical schools helped them prepare for the influx of students pursuing generalist careers once managed care began creating jobs for primary care physicians.

Another example is treatment of people towards the end of their lives. A large research project, called SUPPORT, found that the wishes of dying patients and their families were not being understood by physicians because of difficulties in communication. This disturbing finding led the Foundation to undertake a major multiyear effort to raise the consciousness of the medical profession and the public about the importance of improving the treatment of people towards the end of their lives.

The Robert Wood Johnson Foundation also helps shape public attitudes through its research and communications efforts. Much of what the public knows about the uninsured comes from the widespread distribution of findings from a series of Foundation-funded access-to-care surveys beginning back in 1976. Similarly, much of what is known about medical malpractice, managed care, substance abuse, and sexuality derives from the dissemination of research undertaken by Foundation grantees.

4. Changing the Focus of Demonstration Programs

For its first 15 to 20 years, The Robert Wood Johnson Foundation followed a relatively straightforward strategy. It would often fund a demonstration program that tested an innovative service approach or policy idea in a number of locations; if the approach appeared successful, the federal government would likely take it on and expand it substantially. The early reputation of the Foundation was built upon its national demonstration programs, some of which—emergency medical services and nurse-practitioner training are but two examples—were adopted by the federal government. But the federal government no longer picks up and expands many programs, particularly when these programs increase taxes. As a result, The Robert Wood Johnson Foundation has adopted new and more nuanced approaches to demonstration projects:

- Demonstrations now tend to be larger as the Foundation tries to affect the lives of more people through its programs. As Sharon Begley and Ruby Hearn point out in this volume, the Urban Health Initiative is not just a pilot project. It attempts to improve the health and safety of young people across *entire cities.*

- To a greater extent than before, the Foundation works with state and local governments. Since 1991, for example, it has assisted state governments interested in reforming the financing of health care services. And since 1992, it has supported Making the Grade, a program built on the premise that the long-term financial stability of school-based health services "must be secured through state and community involvement."[3]

- The Foundation now looks to fund coalitions of nongovernmental organizations. One example is the Faith in Action program in which the Foundation supports coalitions of religious congregations and organizations whose members volunteer their services to help those in need. This approach has proved so promising that the Foundation recently agreed to award more than $100 million over the next seven years to fund 2,000 additional local coalitions.

5. Adopting Multi-Faceted Approaches that Embrace Institutions and Fields

In his chapter for this year's *Anthology,* Frank Karel observes, "the most powerful way that foundations can spark social change is to use their monies to fund the creation of new institutions or fundamental change of existing institutions." Although foundations are more limited in their ability to do this than in earlier days, The Robert Wood Johnson Foundation has had a rich experience in developing new institutions and transforming existing ones. With this approach— what might be called "360 degree funding"—all the key aspects of an innovation are covered.

For example, to develop and shape the new profession of nurse-practitioner in the 1970s and 1980s, the Foundation funded nurse-practitioner programs in nursing schools willing to add them; a fellowship program for nurses who became the nucleus of trainers of nurse-practitioners; the creation of a professional society for nurse practitioners; research on relevant aspects of nursing; programs that employed nurse-practitioners, and collaborations among institutions (such as universities, HMOs, state agencies, and employers) to train nurse-practitioners.

Similarly, the Foundation has adopted a wide variety of strategies to encourage managed care organizations to improve the diagnosis and treatment of their members with chronic conditions. It has supported the collection and dissemination of information on HMOs and chronic care; brought together researchers and practitioners focusing on the topic; worked with a national accrediting agency to include chronic care among its indicators; funded demonstration projects; and financed research. While it is too soon to know whether managed care will significantly alter its chronic care practices, this array of programs prepares the groundwork for such institutional change.

6. Reforming Systems of Delivering Health Care Services

Another grantmaking insight derives from the Foundation's many years of experience with programs seeking to overcome the fragmentation of health care services and to reorganize the systems that deliver them. There is much to be learned from its successes and its failures.

First, although "systems change" has a neutral ring to it, systems are rooted in politics and people. What is logical organizational reform for one person may be loss of turf and income for another. Reforming delivery systems implies that foundations understand, and become involved—to some degree at least—in the messiness and factionalism of political processes. As Beth Stevens and Lawrence Brown observe in their chapter in the 1997 *Anthology*, successful interventions require "a systematic reading of the political complexion . . . and close contemplation of the main players in the reform 'game' in terms of the depth of conflicts among their values and interests and the prospects that they might endorse an intervention that they can implement effectively."[4] Foundations have not generally shown an aptitude for this, and, moreover, legal strictures limit what they can do in the governmental arena.

Beyond ascertaining the politics and the players, systems reforms require an understanding of a complex web of laws and regulations. Attempts to provide a seamless net of health care services for home-less people in the Homeless Families Program foundered, in part, on the number and the complexity of the systems that needed to be reformed. Similarly, a national program to integrate acute and long-term care for older people not only had to shape multiple delivery systems but also to coordinate two distinct and complicated government programs, Medicare and Medicaid. In a classic understatement, Joseph Alper and Rosemary Gibson observe in their chapter for this year's *Anthology* that "making the financing of acute and long-term care more rational has proven to be challenging."

Although systems change may be important, it should not be viewed as a panacea. Beginning in 1987, the Foundation funded a series of programs to integrate services for people with chronic mental illness. While the programs were able to change the way mental health services were organized and delivered in some communities, improved service delivery did not necessarily lead to improved mental health. Rather, the emphasis on improving delivery systems obscured the importance of improving the quality of the services themselves. In other words, inadequate services were being delivered in a more efficient manner.

7. Investing in People

One consistent insight emerging from the *Anthology* series is the importance of investing in people in order to bring about long-term improvements in the health care system. From its earliest days, the Foundation has followed a conscious strategy of building the health care field by improving the capacities of those working in it. Since 1972, the Foundation has been supporting the Clinical Scholars Program, which gives physicians committed to academic careers the opportunity to learn about the management, social, computer, and behavioral sciences, and the Health Policy Fellowships Program, which gives mid-career health professionals the opportunity to learn about federal health policy processes by working for a year in a Congressional office. Since the

1980s, its Minority Medical Education Program has been giving qualified minority college students the tools to become better medical school
applicants, and its Minority Medical Faculty Development Program has
been offering research fellowships and mentoring to promising minority junior medical school faculty members. For more than two decades,
the Foundation has supported David Olds, whose research has demonstrated the value of having nurses visit pregnant women in their homes.

Although the notion is difficult to prove, the Foundation's fellowship programs—and others that invest in individuals—are widely considered to be among its successes. They give capable people the
wherewithal to take risks and develop their abilities. As Lewis Sandy
and Richard Reynolds concluded in their analysis of academic medical centers in last year's *Anthology,* "Investments in people pay off
. . . Supporting bright young people early in their career may be
a more effective institutional change strategy than direct institutional
grants."[5] Their conclusion—expanded to include individuals of
all ages—has been echoed throughout the *Anthology* series.

8. Staying in for the Long Run

In its earlier years, the Foundation tended to support programs for a
limited number of years and then move on to other endeavors. While
this approach had the advantage of allowing the Foundation to get
things started and then let others—usually the federal government—
take them over, it also had the potential disadvantage of a premature
exit. Authors of *Anthology* chapters have questioned whether the
Foundation moved away from nurse practitioners, public health dentistry, and regional perinatal programs too early. While nobody can
reasonably expect that a program be continued forever, The Robert
Wood Johnson Foundation now takes a longer-term view, in many
cases supporting programs for a decade or more. This gives institutions and individuals the chance to reach a level of maturity that they
might otherwise not have been able to reach.

9. Maintaining Flexibility

Even with the security given them by longer funding cycles, programs
need to adapt to changing circumstances. Market forces have altered
the course of many Foundation-funded programs: for example, the
Reach Out program to encourage physicians to volunteer their services began just as managed care reduced the free time of doctors, and

the Strengthening Hospital Nursing program attempted to increase hospital nurses' responsibilities at a time when managed care was placing their very jobs in jeopardy. Grantees have had to show great ingenuity just to keep programs alive.

The mercurial nature of the health care system affects the Foundation's strategies as well. Take the evolution of its approach to managed care. As Janet Firshein and Lewis Sandy observe later in this *Anthology*, the Foundation was an early supporter of the nonprofit, staff-driven HMO model that was developing in the 1970s and early 1980s. As a for-profit entrepreneurial model came to dominate managed care in the 1980s and 1990s, the Foundation's approach evolved toward emphasizing quality control in HMOs, encouraging HMOs to provide services for people with chronic illnesses and addictions to tobacco and alcohol, and understanding better the effects of managed care.

10. Respect for Grantees and Ownership of Programs

The tenth and final lesson from the *Anthology* series is the importance of treating grantees and potential grantees with respect, involving them from the early stages of project development, and encouraging program ownership.

In their attempt to discover why some Foundation-supported programs to improve children's health seem to take hold and others do not, Sharon Begley and Ruby Hearn conclude that community ownership is a critical factor. "Without a feeling that a community is guiding a program, there is no public pressure to continue once the Foundation ends its support," they observe. Irene Wielawski noted in last year's *Anthology* that the Local Initiative Funding Partners Program began as one in which The Robert Wood Johnson Foundation exercised considerable power over local foundations. In response to the dissatisfaction this attitude caused among the local foundations, The Robert Wood Johnson Foundation adopted an approach based on mutually respectful relationships among the partners.[6]

The Robert Wood Johnson Foundation often determines its strategic priorities and program designs after extensive consultations with experts. For national programs, it issues a "call for proposals" to which potential applicants are invited to respond. At the same time, the Foundation often holds workshops and meetings with potential applicants, whose ideas are worked into the process even after a call for proposals has been issued. Programs are carried out by the grantees, usually with monitoring and technical support from a national program office and counsel from a national advisory committee of prominent experts. At its best, this process creates a close and mutually respectful relationship between the Foundation and its grantees; enriches the processes and context where innovative ideas are generated, funded, evolved, and developed; and gives grantees ownership of their programs.

In today's hyper-economy, with philanthropic resources surging and new foundations dotting the landscape, it is more important than ever that grant makers share their experiences and learn from one another. The approaches pursued by The Robert Wood Johnson Foundation offer one window into promoting social change in a complex environment. While all foundations are different and there is not necessarily a right way to practice the craft of philanthropy, we hope the *Anthology* series is, and will continue to be, a place to look for insights that readers can adapt to their own circumstances.

San Francisco   Stephen L. Isaacs
Princeton, New Jersey   James R. Knickman
August 2000   Editors

Notes

1. S. A. Schroeder. "Core Values of The Robert Wood Johnson Foundation." In S. L. Isaacs and J. R. Knickman, (eds.), *To Improve Health and Health Care 1998–1999: The Robert Wood Johnson Foundation.* San Francisco: Jossey-Bass, 1998.
2. See chapter 1 by J. M. McGinnis and S. A. Schroeder in this *Anthology.*
3. P. Brodeur. "School-Based Health Clinics." In S. L. Isaacs and J. R. Knickman (eds.), *To Improve Health and Health Care 2000: The Robert Wood Johnson Foundation Anthology.* San Francisco: Jossey-Bass, 1999, p. 14.
4. B. Stevens and L. Brown, "Expertise Meets Politics: Efforts to Work with States." In S. L. Isaacs and J. R. Knickman (eds.), *To Improve Health and Health Care 1997: The Robert Wood Johnson Foundation Anthology.* San Francisco: Jossey-Bass, 1997.
5. L. Sandy and R. Reynolds. "Influencing Academic Health Centers: The Robert Wood Johnson Foundation Experience." In S. L. Isaacs and J. R. Knickman (eds.), *To Improve Health and Health Care 1998–1999: The*

Robert Wood Johnson Foundation Anthology. San Francisco: Jossey-Bass, 1998.

6. I. Wielawski. "The Local Initiative Funding Partners Program." In S. L. Isaacs and J. R. Knickman(eds.), *To Improve Health and Health Care 2000: The Robert Wood Johnson Foundation Anthology.* San Francisco: Jossey-Bass, 1999.

⟶ Acknowledgments

Editing *To Improve Health and Health Care 2001: The Robert Wood Johnson Foundation Anthology* has been a great pleasure in large part because of the excellent team with whom we worked. Most have been colleagues in this endeavor for all four *Anthology* volumes, and we would like to acknowledge their contribution.

If books had godparents, Frank Karel would be the godfather of the *Anthology* series. In addition to writing a fascinating memoir that appears later in this volume, he continued to offer guidance and share his wisdom at all stages of the process.

William Morrill, Patricia Patrizi, and Jonathan Showstack formed the committee that reviewed each manuscript. Their insights and thoughtful analysis greatly strengthened this *Anthology*. C. P. Crow improved the quality of writing and the style of this *Anthology* as he has for each of the previous volumes; his contribution was immeasurable. Molly McKaughan brought her intimate knowledge of the Foundation's programs and her editor's touch to bear in enriching each of the chapters. Richard Toth and Julia Painter reviewed dates and dollars for accuracy and corrected them where necessary—a role that gives us a great feeling of security. Hinda Feige Greenberg worked miracles in finding even the most obscure documents. Deborah Malloy and Sherry Georgianna were invaluable in handling administrative matters within The Robert Wood Johnson Foundation. Linda Potts oversaw with great aplomb the contract under which the *Anthology* was produced, and Joseph Wechselberger was rapid and responsible in his financial analyses. Emily Snell provided valuable research assistance and graphic skills.

Andy Pasternak, Gigi Mark, and Amy Scott at Jossey-Bass made the book's production seem easy. Ty Baldwin entered the edited material, and Chris Chang served as our fact-checker; our thanks to both. We would also like to express appreciation to Susan Hassmiller, Paul

Jellinek, Terrance Keenan, Beth Mastin, Denis Prager, Mark Sachs, Lewis Sandy, Steven Schroeder, Gloria Smith, and Victoria Weisfeld for their review of chapter drafts.

Finally, we owe a special debt of gratitude for the outstanding contribution of John Rodgers, the research and editorial associate for the *Anthology* series. John showed himself to be a consummate professional as he guided the book from idea stage through publication—and still managed to find time to co-author a chapter. His impact on the quality of the book cannot be overstated.

S.L.I.
J.R.K.

To Improve Health and Health Care 2001

Inside the Foundation

—ᴧᴧᴧ— Expanding the Focus of The Robert Wood Johnson Foundation

Health as an Equal Partner to Health Care

J. Michael McGinnis and Steven A. Schroeder

Editors' Introduction

A 1993 article in the *Journal of the American Medical Association* by J. Michael McGinnis and William Foege estimated that more than 40 percent of all deaths in the United States could be attributed to behavior-related causes. For example, the authors attributed 400,000 deaths in 1990 to tobacco, 300,000 to diet and activity patterns, and 100,000 to alcohol. This widely cited article served to wake up many in the health field to the fact that medical care alone can not always ensure better health, nor is it a dominant determinant of health status. It was among the factors that led the Foundation to reconsider its priorities and, in 1999, to make an important change in its focus.

This chapter offers a detailed examination of why and how the Foundation moved from an approach focusing largely on improving health care services to one that gives equal importance to addressing the behavioral and social causes of poor health. It explores the ramifications of this shift—including the largest-ever reorganization of the Foundation's staff into two groups, one focused on health care, the other on health. Additionally, it lays out a blueprint for a grant making program that is currently being developed by the health group.

The authors are well positioned to provide an insiders' view of this change in the Foundation's priorities. Steven A. Schroeder is the president and chief executive officer of The Robert Wood Johnson Foundation. J. Michael McGinnis, the co-author of the 1993 article that helped trigger the change, was named a senior vice-president of the Foundation in 1999. He is the director of the Foundation's health group.

This is the latest in a series of chapters in the *Anthology* series in which senior executives of The Robert Wood Johnson Foundation explain how the Foundation sets priorities and makes funding decisions. In the 1998–99 *Anthology*, Robert Hughes explained the process that led the Foundation's trustees to adopt substance abuse prevention and treatment as a Foundation goal. In that same volume, Steven Schroeder discussed the core values that guide the Foundation's grant making. In the 2000 *Anthology*, James Knickman described priority setting in Foundation-supported research and, in a chapter that appears in this *Anthology*, Frank Karel details the Foundation's strategies in the communications area. Viewed as a whole, these chapters take some of the mystery out of the seemingly impenetrable world of philanthropy.

A t the founding of The Robert Wood Johnson Foundation, its mission was clearly and simply stated: to improve the health and health care of all Americans. Throughout its existence it has been the largest philanthropy devoted exclusively to this field. Yet for much of its first twenty years the Foundation attended predominantly to the medical care element of its mission.[1] That is, it focused on health care delivery, with special emphasis on providing medical services—the *health care* dimension of its mission. By contrast, it neglected the non–medical care factors that influence a person's health, such as choices about smoking, diet, sexual behavior, and physical activity, as well as environmental exposures and other factors— the *health* dimension of its mission.

Over the most recent decade, a shift occurred, first with the incorporation of a major emphasis on substance abuse as a primary source of preventable illness and injury among Americans, and, in 1999, with the decision by the Robert Wood Johnson board of trustees to give formal standing to the health dimension. Today, the Foundation consists of two distinct, overlapping, and roughly equivalent program groups—health and health care. How and why did this evolution occur, and what are its implications?

Early Emphasis on Medical Care

That the early emphasis was on medical care is not surprising. The Foundation's endowment derived from Robert Wood Johnson, who made his family's business, Johnson & Johnson, pre-eminent in the manufacture of medical supplies, devices, and pharmaceuticals; the Foundation's founding president, David Rogers, was a physician and a former medical school dean; and it was created in 1972, as the establishment of Medicare and Medicaid was beginning to funnel tremendous resources and influence into medical care and before the political and medical communities fully realized that many health problems could be prevented. Moreover, the speed of such substantial changes in health financing gave an aura of inevitability to the advent of national health insurance, and instilled some urgency to the idea of increasing the capacity of health care delivery to accommodate the anticipated demand.

During the 1970s and 1980s, however, it became increasingly obvious that the situation was not so simple. National health insurance proved elusive. Indeed, as a result of the formidable political, social, and economic barriers to expanding health insurance coverage, a greater percentage of Americans had health insurance three decades ago, when the Foundation was established, than have it now.[2,3] The Foundation maintained its faithfulness to the principle of better and more equitable insurance coverage, but new concerns arose. The development and the application of new diagnostic and therapeutic technologies, combined with the expanded capacity of the health care system, generated a rapid increase in health care costs, raising the specter of unaffordable care and accentuating the disadvantage for those who were uninsured.

As a proportion of the Gross Domestic Product, medical care costs nearly doubled in the two decades of the 70s and 80s, increasing from 7.4 percent of gross domestic product in 1970 to 13.6 percent in 1992. This alarmed health policy makers and the business community alike; medical cost containment supplanted health insurance expansion as the nation's number one health policy concern and prompted a shift in The Robert Wood Johnson Foundation's concerns away from expanding health care supply to constraining it. The Foundation joined, and even led, elements of the health policy community in exploring and testing attempts to stem the growing costs. These efforts were largely unsuccessful in the near term but offered interesting insights into the entrepreneurial nature of the health delivery and health financing structures that had evolved.[4]

—– Early Steps in Health

While The Robert Wood Johnson Foundation's funding focused on the medical care system, scientific evidence was accumulating to show that medical care was only one of many contributors to personal and national health status.[5,6] Though the United States was the acknowledged world leader in its supply of sophisticated medical technologies for diagnosis and treatment, it lagged far behind other developed countries in traditional health status measures such as infant and maternal mortality rates and life expectancy from birth. Some of that gap reflected limited access to medical care among the poor and the uninsured, but much of the difference was due to factors that lay outside traditional health care delivery—genetic predispositions, social circumstances, physical environments, and behavioral choices (see Figure 1.1 below).

In the mid to late 1980s, several programs were initiated at The Robert Wood Johnson Foundation that transcended the traditional health care boundaries of Foundation support. One, the Infant Health and Development Program, tested whether supportive services to vulnerable infants and their parents could improve subsequent health and educational status. Another tested the impact of home visits by nurses. In contrast to those in comparison groups, 15-year-olds who had been born to unmarried teens in poverty who had received nurse home visits during pregnancy and after birth reported substantially lower rates—often half or less—of arrests, of convictions, of lifetime sex partners, of cigarettes smoked per day, and of days having consumed alcohol in the last six months.[7]

Other programs, such as funding for Fighting Back, a multi-community effort to combat drug abuse and alcoholism, and the Partnership for a Drug-Free America, a media campaign to make illicit drug

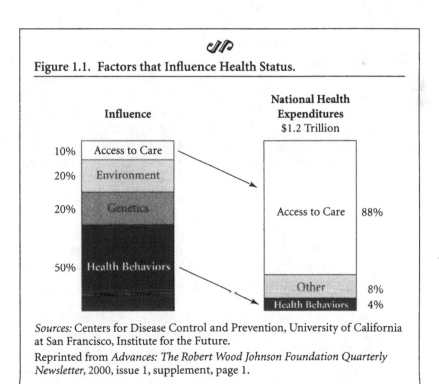

Figure 1.1. Factors that Influence Health Status.

Influence

National Health
Expenditures
$1.2 Trillion

10%	Access to Care
20%	Environment
20%	Genetics
50%	Health Behaviors

Access to Care	88%
Other	8%
Health Behaviors	4%

Sources: Centers for Disease Control and Prevention, University of California at San Francisco, Institute for the Future.

Reprinted from *Advances: The Robert Wood Johnson Foundation Quarterly Newsletter,* 2000, issue 1, supplement, page 1.

use socially unacceptable, extended the Foundation's field of interest directly into near-term efforts to reduce risky behavior. The Foundation's willingness to address the prevention of AIDS also mandated attention to behavioral issues of sexuality and drug use.

As a result of these early programs, in 1988, when the Foundation articulated three new target priorities and ten specific new areas of interest, health issues became a priority for the first time—albeit a relatively low priority. The inclusion of "destructive behavior including drug and alcohol abuse, and mental illness" within the ten areas of specific interest opened the door for more expansive grant making in health. Still notable by its omission was the problem of tobacco use, which contributed more to mortality than alcohol and drug abuse combined.[8]

—— Combating Substance Abuse as a Foundation Goal

With the recruitment in 1990 of a new Robert Wood Johnson Foundation president, Steven A. Schroeder, who was committed to public health and prevention and with a mandate from the trustees to reconsider grant making priorities, the Foundation began a sustained effort to stop the damage caused by harmful substances, including tobacco. Substance abuse seemed an appropriate focus for several reasons. A base of experience had been established through the Foundation's early work in the area. Other foundations had limited involvement with relatively narrow components of the problem, but their support and their programming in this area were negligible. Government activities in the areas of tobacco and alcohol were often politically constrained because of the influence of powerful industry groups. Most important, the evidence about the medical and social damage caused by these substances was irrefutable and compelling.

The program emphasis on substance abuse generated considerable internal debate at the Foundation. Initially, most Robert Wood Johnson staff members were more supportive of developing antidrug programs than of efforts to combat alcohol and tobacco abuse. There was widespread press attention and popular concern about the impact of illegal drugs on society, the federal government had created a drug czar to lead the national assault, and there was no ambiguity about either the pernicious nature of the problem or the politics involved. On the other hand, grant making related to alcohol was complicated by emerging evidence that people who drank in moderation might have better health outcomes than either heavy users or abstainers. And with respect to tobacco, many felt that the antitobacco war had already been won, rendering Foundation support irrelevant.

At a special retreat held in February, 1991, three proposed new goals—targeting substance abuse, access to care, and care for chronic conditions—were brought forward for consideration of the trustees. Only the substance abuse goal received much debate, and the trustees quickly found themselves at an impasse. While all agreed that the public health case was strong, there was substantial debate about becoming involved in tobacco and alcohol. Proponents argued that it would appear hypocritical to limit the focus to the issue of illicit drugs, given that the toll from tobacco and alcohol was so much higher. Opponents countered that tobacco and alcohol were legal substances, that people had the right to choose whether and to what degree to use those substances, and that controversy would result from the inevitable conflict with the powerful tobacco and alcohol industries.[9] A compromise was reached whereby all three types of substances would be included, with initial programs aimed at tobacco and alcohol use directed only at children and young people, for whom these substances were illegal. Thus, for the first time a *health* topic emerged as a separate Robert Wood Johnson program goal, and grant making in the substance abuse area flourished over the next decade.

After early experience with grants aimed at reducing youth exposure to tobacco and alcohol, the target age group gradually expanded to include binge drinking by college students, tobacco cessation for adults in managed care, state coalitions against tobacco use, and other substance abuse efforts. The issues debated in the 1991 board retreat have often resurfaced in subsequent discussions among both staff members and trustees: tensions between public health and civil liberties; the role of government in safeguarding the health of the public, especially young people; and the Foundation's role *vis-a-vis* industry. Nevertheless, over time the Foundation clearly became more comfortable with grant making in this arena, solidified its original sense that philanthropic efforts in substance abuse had great potential to improve the health of the public, and was able to enlist other foundations and organizations to join with it.

A notable example was the start-up of the National Center for Tobacco-Free Kids in 1996. The Foundation and the American Cancer Society were the two major founding sponsors, and they were joined by the Annie E. Casey Foundation, the Conrad Hilton Foundation, the Henry Ford Health System, the Henry J. Kaiser Family Foundation, the American Heart Association, and the American Medical Association in the effort. Concurrently, the national attitude toward the tobacco industry was also shifting, in part because of other developments such as the release of industry documents about concealment of intent, the successful litigation strategies of state attorneys general, and scientific evidence demonstrating changes in the brains of addicted smokers, paralleling similar changes in drug addicts.

As people recognized not only the importance of this issue in general but also the Foundation's leadership in particular, staff and board concerns were replaced by pride at the Foundation's contributions to preventing substance abuse. By the end of 1999, the Foundation's active commitments for substance abuse amounted to $361 million or 27 percent of all of its commitments at that time, and substance abuse was clearly established as a crucial part of the Foundation's sphere of interest. For the period January 1972 through December 1999, the Foundation's total commitment in substance abuse equaled $820 million in both active and closed programs.

—— Establishment of Health as a Full Partner with Health Care

Coincident with the evolution of programming in substance abuse as a clear and central focus for the Foundation's agenda, evidence was accumulating that future improvements in health status were more likely to come from influences outside the medical care domain.[10,11,12,13,14] Epidemiological studies that were begun with the rapid growth in the National Institutes of Health in the 1950s and 1960s generated important insights in the 1970s and 1980s on the role of a variety of behavioral factors underlying the nation's leading killers—heart and lung disease, cancer, stroke, diabetes. Findings from environmental and occupational studies identified several serious long-term effects from exposure to a variety of environmental toxins, including lead, asbestos, radon, mercury, polychlorinated biphenyls (PCBs), nitrates, and certain atmospheric pollutants. Work in genetics offered increasing evidence on human biological predispositions to certain diseases, and vulnerabilities to behavioral and environmental exposures. Interesting hints began to emerge in the 1980s and 1990s of pathways by which the stress of social circumstances might affect susceptibility to certain diseases. As understanding deepened regarding the origins of and vulnerability to disease, additional opportunities emerged for broader health initiatives that had the potential to make a difference in the health of Americans.

As knowledge was growing, so were the Foundation's resources. Because of the sustained bull market of the 1990s, the Foundation's assets—and thus the size of its grant making—grew at a rapid pace, climbing from $2.6 billion in 1990 to $6.7 billion by the start of 1998. It became apparent that the increased growth was stretching the Foundation in several ways. First, although staff growth lagged significantly behind asset growth, the sheer number of professional staff members made the old collegial style of everyone's sitting around a table and debating proposed programs less tenable. This was symbolized physically by the fact that we outgrew our meeting room. Second, the previous structures and processes that governed grant formation and oversight were in danger of breaking down under the increased workload. In addition, it became evident that the Foundation could benefit from bringing on staff with special expertise, such as health care financing or treatment of alcoholism. Yet the old organizational format was not ideally aligned for such specialized recruiting, because it lacked specific objectives. Furthermore, a reorganization might provide new opportunities to improve the strategic focus of grant making.

In January 1997, the President's Message to the trustees signaled that change might be necessary to accommodate the Foundation's growth. It seemed appropriate to accommodate growth by investing further in grant making in health, because the Foundation's experience to date had been so positive and the evidence of possible return so compelling. Given the growth in assets, it appeared that the Foundation could have its cake and eat it too—that is, it could retain its traditional emphasis on health care delivery while at the same time moving toward parity in its health grant making. The message prompted a great deal of discussion among the trustees and staff about the issues and possible approaches. For example, the possibility of creating a sub-foundation—located in another city—that would specialize in substance abuse was seriously explored. Such a move would relieve the problem of overcrowding and provide an interesting model of decentralized and focused grant making. Over the next two years, staff members and trustees held meetings, interviews, and planning sessions to consider the various options. The trustees rejected the idea of a stand-alone substance abuse foundation because they were more comfortable with the tighter governance model provided by having all programs and staff under the same roof. Instead, they adopted a different form of decentralization: the Foundation reorganized into two distinct but overlapping groups, or clusters of staff interested in kindred issues, one to focus on health and the other on health care. This reorganization established health as an equal partner with health care for the first time. A national search was conducted for leaders of the two groups, and in the spring of 1999, two new senior vice presidents were appointed. Jack Ebeler was brought in to direct the Health Care Group, and J. Michael McGinnis to direct the Health Group.

⎯ An Agenda for Health

Throughout 1999, the Health Group worked to identify those areas where Foundation leadership and investment could best influence the health of the general population. Because even a foundation the size and reach of The Robert Wood Johnson Foundation could not reasonably expect to provide leadership in all the areas that influence health status, the immediate challenge has been to identify those that present the greatest opportunities for the Foundation at this time. Three criteria have helped guide our choices: addressing the problems of greatest importance to the health of Americans; building on the strengths and experience of The Robert Wood Johnson Foundation in philanthropy; and working in ways in which Foundation leadership might make the most lasting contribution to building the field of population-wide health improvement.

Addressing Problems of Greatest Importance to Americans' Health

The primary influence that stands out as a critical controllable determinant of the health of Americans is behavior. Behavioral factors have been estimated to account for more than 40 percent of deaths among Americans, with the most prominent contributions coming from tobacco, patterns of diet and physical activity, alcohol, risky sexual behavior, use of guns, drug use, and operation of motor vehicles. The first three of these alone account for about a third of all deaths.[15]

Social circumstances are also a major determinant of health. Educational level, poverty, and race all contribute to health disparities. Among people aged 25 to 64 years in the United States, the overall death rate for those with less than 12 years of education is twice that of people with 13 or more years of education.[16] People in poverty have about a one-third higher risk of dying in any given year than those in the general population.[17] Even after adjusting for tobacco and alcohol use, obesity and physical activity levels, people who have sustained economic hardship for long periods are nearly three times more likely to be disabled than those who have not sustained such economic hardships.[18] Relative to other Americans, African Americans are more likely to die in infancy, the teen years, and adulthood.[19] People who perceive themselves to be socially isolated—that is, who feel particularly disadvantaged or estranged from others in society as a result of economic, geographic, cultural, or other personal circumstances—report added stress and often have two to three times the risk of health problems.[20] How people view their place in society may also work to increase their risk.[21]

The physical environment is also important to health prospects. Some of our greatest health gains have come as a result of improvements in the quality and the safety of our water, air, and food supplies. On balance, the safeguards in these areas are working reasonably well. The principal challenges from our physical environments are twofold: maintaining our capacity and our vigilance to safeguard water, air, and food; and understanding and monitoring the influence of global factors—such as climate change, atmospheric pollution, and infectious diseases emerging in new places as a result of ecosystem change—that will shape the magnitude of the environment's influence on our health.

Genetics is another area of increasing importance to health. Although purely genetic diseases are rare and of limited impact on the health of the entire population, developments from the human genome project can be expected to add to the capacity to target preventive interventions for individuals and populations at greatest risk. The important issue is not how much disease and disability is caused by genetic aberrations but how genetically determined susceptibilities interact with environment, behavior, and social conditions to bring on disease.

Building on Our Strengths

As we explored ways to build on the established record of the Foundation, three areas where the Foundation had relevant experience emerged: the experience gained in substance abuse; that gained in working in communities to reach disadvantaged populations; and that gained through leadership development programs such as the Clinical Scholars Program that draw the best and brightest professionals at the postdoctoral level into fields they might not otherwise have had the opportunity to explore.

- Substance abuse

  The fact that the Foundation had, at the time of the reorganization, a decade of programming targeted on substance abuse offered an important base on which to build, offering lessons about the challenges of effecting behavior change. Although the Foundation's work in substance abuse has helped to attract new leadership and policy initiative to the field, and has provided the platform for cooperative work among key parties, the task is far from complete. Tobacco, alcohol, and illicit drug use still drain the nation's health and productivity.

- Community initiatives

  Many activities launched with Foundation support, both related to substance abuse and to improving access to medical services among those in need, have focused on work and change at the community level. The Foundation has devoted substantial investment to better understanding community dynamics, leadership processes, and agents of change in its efforts.

- Leadership

  Among the Foundation's most visible, long-standing, and successful contributions have been its initiatives to attract and train a new generation of leaders in health policy. Because the beginning days of the Foundation's existence coincided with the early days of the dramatic explosion of issues related to health services financing and delivery—a time in which the ranks for analytic and policy leadership in the field were very thin, and virtually nonexistent among the medical community—the Foundation's Clinical Scholars Program, the Scholars in Health Policy Research, the Investigator Awards in Health Policy Research, and the Executive Nurse Fellows Program have all filled important gaps in the nation's capacity for thought and leadership.[22]

Opportunities To Make a Lasting Contribution

In a way, a similar opportunity now exists for creative thought and policy leadership for population-wide strategies for health improvement. A new field of population health is emerging, a field that addresses the root causes of disease and disability—identifies them, characterizes them, and intervenes against them through clustered programs—and, by doing so, seeks an allocation of social resources for health improvement that is both more effective and more efficient.

To design and implement our contributions to the health field, we have chosen to structure the activities of the Health Group around five teams: tobacco; alcohol and illegal drugs; health and behavior, with a special emphasis on physical activity; community health, with emphasis on social connectedness; and population health science and policy. We have chosen tobacco, alcohol, and illegal drugs as priorities because they represent the most pronounced influence on early death, disability, and dysfunction among Americans, and because the Foundation has developed a strong record of leadership in the field. We have chosen physical activity as a priority because we now know it is a matter of vital importance to the health of every American, the prevailing trends have been in the wrong direction for a generation and because no alternative sources of national leadership with substantial resources to address the problem exist. We have chosen community health and a focus on socially isolated populations, both because of the need for more understanding and action in the area and because the Foundation has a long record of community-based programs. And we have chosen population health because the field is in its infancy and requires resources devoted to research and policy development in order to build it.

The Teams of the Health Group

Tobacco

The tobacco team seeks to decrease the number of Americans who use tobacco. We have a well-established and active agenda of current programs in tobacco.[23] A special opportunity is offered to the field of tobacco control with monies now available through the states' tobacco settlement, so The Robert Wood Johnson Foundation will now focus on preventing tobacco use by stimulating stronger state and federal policy actions and helping addicted tobacco users quit by promoting the use of effective treatments.

Alcohol and Illegal Drugs

The alcohol and illegal drugs team aims to reduce the negative health and social consequences that abuse of alcohol and illegal drugs has on people. Over the last decade, the Foundation has provided leadership on and visibility for the issue of substance abuse.[24] One of the principal shortfalls remains the failure to apply appropriate treatment, despite increasing evidence of the effectiveness of treatment protocols. The combination of target populations that are hard to reach, society's natural aversion to drug addicts, payment systems that do not include substance abuse treatment as a part of routine medical care, and a lack of professional interest in confronting substance abuse problems make this an especially challenging and important problem.

Health and Behavior

The health and behavior team is attempting to increase Americans' healthy behavior, especially physical activity. Health-related behavior change is not a new focus for the Foundation—many substance abuse programs have focused on behavior change—but the emphasis on physical activity does represent a new departure. Information from epidemiological studies conducted over the last decade offers powerful testimony about the importance of physical activity across the life span in protecting against a variety of health problems. Compared to earlier generations in which work and living styles were more active, our population has become increasingly sedentary; in 1997, 40 percent of adults performed no leisure time physical activity at all.[25] Producing even small changes in activity levels might yield major health benefits. The Foundation, therefore, is supporting efforts to bring physical activity back into Americans' lives, and specifically hopes to increase the activity levels of sedentary middle-aged and older adults. In the broader arena of health behavior, the Foundation is seeking to promote more attention to these issues by doctors and nurses during the course of routine medical visits.

Community Health

The community health team is addressing the community and social factors that promote individual health, primarily by focusing on bringing those whose social circumstances leave them feeling

estranged from others and at increased risk for adverse health outcomes—such as pregnant teenagers in poverty, juveniles who are
chronically truant or in trouble, or older people living alone—into
better supportive relationships. Although the work of this team
offers a new grouping for community-based activities, the Foundation has long funded community-level health programs. Examples
of such programs include home visiting by nurses, family resource
centers, and interfaith volunteer caregiving. Given the increasing
body of knowledge confirming the importance of strong community ties in enhancing the health prospects of individuals at risk of
social isolation, the community health team is focusing on improving community outreach to socially isolated individuals and understanding better how social support and connectedness can improve
health.

Population Health Science and Policy

The population health science and policy team seeks to promote
knowledge, leadership, and methods of enhancing population-wide
health improvement strategies and programs. In order to achieve the
goal of improving the health of all Americans, the Foundation needs
to make long-term investments that will increase the number of
researchers working to understand factors that promote healthy
lives; it also needs to improve the quality and use of methods that
can measurably improve a community's health. Existing investments
in this area include the Turning Point program that is attempting to
revitalize public health at the state and local levels; an effort, now in
the planning stage, to create a center fostering the application of
commercial marketing techniques for health improvement ("social
marketing"); work to foster improved understanding of the effectiveness of childhood immunization; and a range of programs to
encourage the development of leadership in the public health field.
We envision major initiatives in the coming years to take advantage
of Internet and web-based health information technology for consumers and for public health; to engage highly trained scholars in
issues important to population health; to sponsor centers of
research, analysis, and practice targeted to population health
improvement; and to encourage policy interventions that support
population health improvement.

~~~ Looking Forward: The Promise and Challenges

Expanding our health grant making holds the promise of focusing our attention and resources on the many powerful determinants of health status that lie outside the reach of medical care. As has sometimes happened in the past, by focusing its attention on a field, The Robert Wood Johnson Foundation might spur other foundations, government entities, and the media to give it attention as well. If this happens, the Foundation could be a catalyst in a nationwide effort that results in Americans living healthier lives. Certainly, a shift in priorities that gives as high a place to healthy behaviors as to good medical care would be salutary.

Whether these promises will be realized depends on how well we develop strategies, identify the right initiatives and grantees, and evaluate and communicate the results of programs. This is a major hurdle, one that the program teams are devoting great effort to overcoming. Moreover, the success of these efforts will depend on the extent to which The Robert Wood Johnson Foundation can forge partnerships with other philanthropies and with public agencies. Under the best of circumstances, establishing collaborations is complicated;[26] in an area new to the Foundation, it may be even more challenging.

Another challenge is maintaining focus while we carry out a greatly expanded mandate. While we must stretch our horizons and extend our reach in order to build the nation's capacity to understand, take action, and formulate policies related to health improvement, it is clear that a single foundation cannot do everything. We have limited our health grant making to five discrete areas, albeit broad ones.

The very notion of trying to build a field—in this case the field of population health—carries with it interesting challenges. In philanthropy, we often think of ourselves as seeking to enhance the development of a field in one aspect or another—and there have been some discernible successes in that respect. The early contributions of the Rockefeller Foundation to the green revolution that increased global food production come to mind, as do the work of the Carnegie Corporation with libraries and the Ford Foundation with schools of public policy. The Robert Wood Johnson Foundation has gained, over the years, considerable experience in helping to establish and strengthen new fields—from emergency medical services to tobacco policy research. As part of our efforts to develop the field of population health, we will bring to bear the experience of our foundation as well as those of other foundations that have helped establish new fields.

The Foundation's reorganization offers both opportunities and challenges. Under any circumstances, change is difficult; massive change is even more unnerving. In the case of The Robert Wood Johnson Foundation, three changes are taking place simultaneously: a new strategic vision that gives health an equal status with health care; a reorganization of the staff into two groups (with distinct mandates but inevitably overlapping interests) and eleven program management teams; and development of new, quantifiable objectives for each program area. The way in which the Foundation adapts to change and meets the challenges inherent in each of these areas will affect its ability to reach its aspirations and will provide lessons of interest to our colleagues in the philanthropic community.

It is clear that improving the health of the American population will require fundamental changes in human behavior.[27,28] Merely providing more and better access to medical care—as important as that is— will not be sufficient to make us a healthier nation. Nor will investment in basic research alone—as promising as this may be—bring fundamental improvement in the health of our population. Obviously, it is easier to say that improvements in health determinants are essential than it is to make those improvements a reality. Nevertheless, by establishing health as a full and equal partner with health care, The Robert Wood Johnson Foundation has pledged to do its part in pursuing that goal.

Notes

1. R. Hughes. "Adopting the Substance Abuse Goal." In S. L. Isaacs and J. R. Knickman (eds.), *To Improve Health and Health Care 1998–1999: The Robert Wood Johnson Foundation Anthology.* San Francisco: Jossey Bass, 1998, pp. 3–18.

2. S. A. Schroeder. "The Medically Uninsured: Will They Always Be with Us?" *New England Journal of Medicine,* 1996, *334,* 1130–1133.

3. S. A. Schroeder, "President's Message," *The Robert Wood Johnson Foundation 1999 Annual Report.*

4. L. D. Brown and C. McLaughlin. "Constraining Costs at the Community Level: A Critique." *Health Affairs,* 1990, *9*(1): 5–28.

5. J. M. McGinnis and W. H. Foege. "Actual Causes of Death in the United States." *Journal of the American Medical Association,* 1993, *270*(18): 2207–2212.

6. J. M. McGinnis. "United States." In C. Everett Koop, C. E. Pearson, and R. Schwarz (eds.), *Critical Issues in Global Health.* San Francisco: Jossey-Bass, 2001.

7. D. Olds et al. "Long-term Effects of Nurse Home Visitation on Children's Criminal and Antisocial Behavior: 15-Year Follow-up of a Randomized Controlled Trial." *Journal of the American Medical Association,* 1998, *280*(14), 1238–1244.

8. J. M. McGinnis and W. H. Foege. "Actual Causes of Death in the United States." *Journal of the American Medical Association,* 1993, *270*(18), 2207–2212.

9. R. G. Hughes. "Adopting the Substance Abuse Goal: A Story of Philanthropic Decision Making." In S. L. Isaacs and J. R. Knickman, (eds.), *To Improve Health and Health Care 1998–1999: The Robert Wood Johnson Foundation Anthology.* San Francisco: Jossey Bass, 1998, pp. 3–18.

10. J. Knowles. *Doing Better and Feeling Worse: Health in the United States.* New York: Norton, 1977.

11. U.S. Public Health Service. *Healthy People: Surgeon General's Report on Health Promotion and Disease Prevention.* Washington, D.C.: Government Printing Office, 1979.

12. D. A. Hamburg, D. L. Parron, and G. R. Elliott. *Health and Behavior: Frontiers of Research in the Biobehavioral Sciences.* Washington D.C.: National Academy Press, 1982.

13. M. Lalonde. *A New Perspective on the Health of Canadians.* Ottawa, Canada: Government of Canada, 1974.

14. G. Rose. *The Strategy of Preventive Medicine.* Oxford: Oxford University Press, 1992.

15. J. M. McGinnis and W. H. Foege. "Actual Causes of Death in the United States." *Journal of the American Medical Association,* 1993, *270*(18), 2207–2212.

16. U.S. Department of Health and Human Services. *Healthy People 2010.* Washington, D.C.: Government Printing Office, 2000.

17. P. D. Sorlie, E. Backlund, and J. B. Keller, "U.S. Mortality by Economic, Demographic, and Social Characteristics: The National Longitudinal Mortality Study." *American Journal of Public Health,* 1995, *85*(7), 949–956.

18. J. W. Lynch et al. "Cumulative Impact of Sustained Economic Hardship on Physical, Cognitive, Psychological, and Social Functioning." *New England Journal of Medicine,* 1997, *337*(26), 1889–1895.

19. Analysis of "United States Life Tables, 1997." National Vital Statistics Report, 1999, 47(28).

20. J. S. House, K. Landis, and D. Umberson. "Social Relationships and Health." *Science,* 1988, *241*(4865), 540–545.

21. S. L. Syme. "Control and Health: A Personal Perspective." in A. Steptoe and A. Appels, (eds.), *Stress, Personal Control and Health.* (London: Wiley, 1989), pp. 3–18.

22. S. L. Isaacs, L. G. Sandy, and S. A. Schroeder. "Improving the Health Care Workforce: Perspectives from Twenty-Four Years' Experience." In S. L. Isaacs and J. R. Knickman, (eds.), *To Improve Health and Health Care 1997: The Robert Wood Johnson Foundation Anthology.* San Francisco: Jossey Bass, 1997, pp. 21–52.

23. These include SmokeLess States to create private sector tobacco control coalitions, Smoke-Free Families and Addressing Tobacco in Managed Care to create new models for tobacco cessation for pregnant women and those served by managed care, the Campaign for Tobacco-Free Kids to change social norms about tobacco use, the Research Network on the Etiology of Tobacco Dependence to better understand the transition from experimental use to addiction in adolescents, the Substance Abuse Policy Research Program to study the effects of tobacco control policies, and the Transdisciplinary Tobacco Use Research Centers to bring researchers from various disciplines together to research difficult problems.

24. It has done this by supporting the National Center on Addiction and Substance Abuse at Columbia University and the Partnership for a Drug-Free America's media campaign; by establishing community coalitions to address substance abuse through Fighting Back and providing support for the national coalition movement through Join Together and Community Anti-Drug Coalitions of America; by supporting research through the Substance Abuse Policy Research Program; by documenting the problem of binge drinking on college campuses through the College Alcohol Survey; and by exploring intervention and treatment opportunities through Screening and Brief Intervention for Alcohol Abuse in Managed Care and Demonstration and Evaluation of Substance Abuse Treatment in Welfare Reform Programs.

25. U.S. Department of Health and Human Services, *Healthy People 2010.* Washington, D.C.: Government Printing Office, 2000.

26. See S. L. Isaacs and J. H. Rodgers, "Partnership Among National Foundations: Between Rhetoric and Reality," in this year's *Anthology.*

27. S. A. Schroeder, "Understanding Health Behavior and Speaking Out on the Uninsured: Two Leadership Opportunities: The 1999 Robert H. Ebert Memorial Lecture." *Academic Medicine,* 1999, *74,* 1163–1171.

28. S. A. Schroeder, "Improving the Health of the American Public Requires a Broad Research Agenda." *Academic Medicine,* 1999, *74,* 530–531.

CHAPTER TWO

—⁓— "Getting the Word Out"
A Foundation Memoir
and Personal Journey

Frank Karel[1]

Editors' Introduction

This chapter is a personal reflection by Frank Karel on his years as vice president for communications of The Robert Wood Johnson Foundation. He looks back on the early days, when the Foundation was groping to find an appropriate role for communications, and traces its evolution to the present. Karel is uniquely qualified to provide this retrospective. He has had the singular experience of heading communications at The Robert Wood Johnson Foundation twice. During his first tenure, between 1974 and 1987, he originated many of the communications strategies that the Foundation follows today. After leaving to head communications at the Rockefeller Foundation, he returned to The Robert Wood Johnson Foundation in 1993 to serve again as the vice president for communications, the position he occupies today. Long active in philanthropy—he is currently a board member of the Council on Foundations—Karel has helped many foundations consider how best to use the tools of communications.

From the beginning, The Robert Wood Johnson Foundation recognized the importance of communications. Starting with a public relations perspective in the 1970s, it evolved to its current state, where communications is an integral component of regular programmatic activities, where communications officers are members of the teams planning and overseeing Foundation-funded initiatives, and where communications has become a major intervention in its own right, accounting for nearly 20 percent of the funds awarded by the Foundation over the past five years. Moreover, the Foundation has been a leader in the nonprofit world in utilizing the channels and techniques of communications—whether through the media, the Internet, social marketing, or its own publications—to advance its mission.

Any nonprofit organization interested in advancing innovation in the field needs to understand and make the most of communications. Getting the word out is essential to bringing about social change. Not only does this chapter provide an informative history of what The Robert Wood Johnson Foundation has done, but it also distills more than 20 years of experience from a person widely recognized as one of the preeminent thinkers and actors in the field.

T he Robert Wood Johnson Foundation has had a long learning curve on the value of information and communications. The first lesson on the power of this combination was in December 1971, the night after it was announced that we were in business as a national philanthropy. The information that a foundation with $1.2 billion was operating out of a small Victorian house in New Brunswick, New Jersey—communicated in a *New York Times* front-page article—was enough to motivate someone to break in and ransack the place before abandoning dreams of misbegotten riches and skulking off with a few office odds and ends.

In truth, the Foundation's first applications of communications *were* driven by the determination to distribute our funds effectively, but as grants rather than loot. We wanted all the people directing institutions and organizations that could become applicants and grantees to know the Foundation existed, what we were willing to fund and what we weren't, and the terms and processes by which an exchange could take place—our funds for their commitment, capacity, and ideas for moving toward a shared objective "to improve the health and health care of all Americans." Carefully shaping these funding guidelines became a priority of the Foundation's initial staff, and our president made this his centerpiece in the Foundation's first annual report as a national philanthropy, which was widely distributed throughout the health sector and the philanthropic community.

Even so, we were an unknown and untested institution in those early days. When we sent out our first announcements of a competitive grant program for the country's community hospitals, we had to include a copy of our *Annual Report* to let the hospital officials know—to communicate—who we were and that we had sufficient funds to be offering sixty $500,000 grants for the establishment of group practices in underserved areas. This past year, we issued 26 such announcements, or Calls for Proposals, but we've become well enough known to skip including an *Annual Report*.

The Formative Years

Foundations have been slower to integrate communications into their institutional planning and work than any other class of organizations in our society. This is not surprising, given a cultural bias with three deep roots: the Judeo-Christian ethic that charity ought to be practiced quietly, avoiding public notice; a widely held conviction that foundation funds are private assets; and another belief that foundation trustees' stewardship is primarily defined by donor intent in establishing the foundation.

Just three years before The Robert Wood Johnson Foundation emerged as a national institution, the Tax Reform Act of 1969 became a federal statute. It still stands as the most sweeping single piece of legislation affecting the operation of private foundations. Because foundations had had a very bad time of it in the congressional hearings leading up to its passage, the prevailing mood and mindset in the foundation world was to keep as quiet and as low a public profile as possible. Even today, that experience continues to affect the view of many foundation officials.

There was an immediate tension between shying away from publicity and the Foundation's commitment to using its funds to further specific goals, initially encapsulated as "the encouragement of institutions or individuals who are attempting to restructure the American health delivery system to make effective care more available for non-hospitalized patients."[2] The first staff members knew that to accomplish this goal they would have to reach widely and deeply into the nation's health sector to find and encourage pioneers, to build alliances, and to design and fund programs—all requiring communications well beyond the norm for foundations.

I believe the convergence of this goal orientation with three other factors caused the Foundation to break from the existing pattern and make communications an integral part of both management and program. First, academic medical centers had been the prior workplace or focus of work for most of Robert Wood Johnson's initial professional staff. These institutions had grown remarkably by communicating the value of biomedical research and the application of its results to the public, especially federal and state policy makers. Carrying this thinking over into the Foundation was a natural step. "We must serve as more accessible sources of information and assistance to those we serve, and find better ways of reporting on the outcome of the endeavors we aid so that more can learn from our experiences," the late David Rogers, the Foundation's first president, wrote in his *Annual Report* message the year I joined the staff to develop a communications program.[3] The chairman of the board of trustees, a formidable, crusty retired Johnson & Johnson executive with a heart of gold who had been hand-picked by Robert Wood Johnson for the job, was more succinct. "Getting the word out" was how the late Gustav O. (Gus) Lienhard used to describe the communications function.

The second factor that caused us to break with the foundation world's pattern of downplaying communications is idiosyncratic and personal, but that's the nature of private foundations. They are largely what one, or two, or a few individuals make them. Rogers and his four principal shapers of the Foundation's initial program—Robert Blendon, the late Walsh McDermott, Margaret Mahoney, and Terrance Keenan—understood the potential value of effective communications through their previous work in the health sectors. Our careers had all crossed and twined in interesting ways. David Rogers had been chairman of the National Advisory Committee for the National Jewish Medical and Research Center, where I was director of planning, when he became the president of the Foundation. He and I had discussed the role that communications might play in a foundation seeking "to help a field move from A to B." Before my arrival I had given Rogers a paper—which he shared with the senior staff—setting out my views on how communications might be harnessed to further the Foundation's objectives. The staff concurred with the approach I outlined, so that even before I arrived, the key players had agreed on the importance of communications to the new Foundation. Moreover, the Foundation's style of group exploration, debate, and resolution ensured me a place at the table where programs were shaped and decisions were made. That my professional background included work as a foundation program officer and institutional planner as well as an institutional communicator—all in the health sector—added to their comfort level with my participation.

The third and final factor influencing us to integrate communications with program and management was a little booklet that has already been mentioned—our *Call for Proposals*. Known internally as the CFP, it is used to announce the Foundation's multisite national programs (those in which grants are made to a number of institutions—from four to as many as 1,100—for research, policy analyses, or training in a particular field, or to support advocacy efforts toward some particular end such as the reduction of youth smoking, or to field test a new way of organizing, delivering, or financing health care services). In the beginning, and even now, the CFP brings the program concepts to life by combining a succinct description of the problems addressed by the program, the elements of the projects that we will fund to overcome them, what is expected of the grantees, and eligibility and selection criteria.

Over the years, creating a CFP has become second nature to communications and program staff alike, but it was not always so. Early on, in addition to developing the format, the communications contribution was to distill notes from scores of meetings and discussions, staff papers, and professional literature into 2,000 or so words that, in terms familiar to the intended audiences of grant applicants, would strike the necessary balances between Foundation and grantee interests and still be clear and compelling.

Even the idea of grant making for communications purposes came early. In 1975, we co-funded a film on hospital-sponsored group practices for use in explaining that concept to the boards and medical staffs of hospitals eligible to apply for grants under one of our multisite national programs. The film producer was a relatively unknown independent named Henry Hampton, who, before he died in 1998, went on to fame as producer of *Eyes on the Prize*, the acclaimed PBS series on the civil rights movement.

A key point, however, is that while this process brought communications staff members into the center of program design and development in the early years, it is only in the last five years that the integration has had large-scale programmatic consequences. In this later period, 19 percent of our grant dollars have supported communications activities.

I vividly remember one of my first conversations with board chairman Gus Lienhard in which he and I found we were in agreement that the Foundation ought to maintain a relatively low public profile, becoming known through the work of its grantees. This concept has been our communications compass for more than a quarter of a century and has emerged as one of the core values of the Foundation. In the words of Steven A. Schroeder, our current president, "We speak through our grantees and do not seek a high institutional profile. We have chosen to work primarily through our grantees, rather than establish ourselves as a primary source of information."[4] This, and the value placed on information by the Foundation, was underscored by including a bibliography of selected books, articles, and other information by our grantees in the 1976 *Annual Report*—a practice that has been broadened to include their work on the Web, video, data tapes, and audio visuals, and continued to this day.

The primacy of program and the principle of speaking through our grantees also shaped a key dimension in the role of the directors of our national programs. Typically, the directors of these programs are highly respected professionals in their fields who remain as employees of their home institutions, directing their programs on a part-time basis with a small staff whose salaries and operations are funded by the Foundation. They, not a Foundation officer, serve as spokespersons for the programs and, when appropriate, on the issues addressed by the programs. Most of the time, this plays out in relatively friendly or benign circumstances—presentations to audiences of other professionals, press interviews, and the like—but not always. The first such departure from the norm came in 1981, when the program director of our School Health Services Program, a Johns Hopkins University faculty member, went to rural Utah for a series of tense meetings with community residents and leaders after a conservative advocacy group began a series of verbal attacks on the local site. Having an outside expert with hands-on experience like, in this instance, Catherine DeAngelis, a pediatrician who put herself through medical school by working as a nurse, goes a long way toward defusing such situations and confirms the wisdom of speaking through our programs and grantees. Today, Dr. DeAngelis is the editor of the *Journal of the American Medical Association*.

That early principle of being known through our grantees has determined the focus and the content of virtually all the Foundation's publications and communications products, other than the *Annual Report*, beginning with a *Special Report* in 1977 on three grant-supported initiatives—a California program training nurse practitioners in rural family practices; new community-based approaches to the prevention and treatment of child abuse and neglect; and a program underwriting staff for the health committees in the legislatures of Connecticut, Louisiana, Michigan, Minnesota, New Jersey, Texas, Washington, and Wyoming. The most unfortunate departures from this principle have been two videos that attempted to explain the Foundation through the work and the processes of our staff. They turned out to be so self-serving that one is used only as an object lesson to avoid this pitfall. The other was banished from sight so successfully that no copy can be found today.

—— Communications Today

Today, communications has become an integral part of everything we do, and in turn we help our grantees integrate communications into their programs. The aim is to share our vision of using communications strategically—that is, to create and use information in ways that can help achieve key organizational and program objectives.

Although every unit of the Foundation is involved to some degree, primary responsibility rests with the Communications Department with its staff of 34 augmented by scores of others engaged for varying

ℐℛ

Table 2.1.   The Robert Wood Johnson Foundation
             Communications Department Mission.

The Communications Department plans and executes activities
creating information and effecting the exchange of information
tailored to foster relationships and actions crucial to advancing
the Foundation's mission and goals.

STRATEGIES

In carrying out its mission—and using grants, contracts, and the direct
efforts of its staff—the Communications Department employs seven
strategies:

1. Working with other Foundation staff in all phases of institutional and
   program planning, as well as in proposal review and development, to
   incorporate provisions for strategic communications.*
2. Helping grantees build their capacities for employing strategic
   communications in their research, evaluation, training, and service-
   demonstration projects and programs for a variety of purposes,
   including:
   • Building and maintaining alliances
   • Raising supplemental funds
   • Recruiting staff and volunteers
   • Creating and maintaining favorable and even supportive media and
     policy climates
   • Disseminating the results and findings of their work
   • Moving issues and solutions into mainstream thinking and
     practice.
3. Making the findings and lessons learned by the Foundation and
   our grantees accessible to other individuals and organizations—
   at national, state, and local levels—that can benefit from this
   information.
4. Encouraging the adoption of health-care innovations and health
   promoting behaviors.

periods of time each year as consultants. In addition to founding the
unit in 1974, I had the privilege of serving as its head until leaving the
Foundation in 1986, resuming that post when I returned to the Foundation in 1993.

The Department's seven strategies for pursuing its mission (see
Table 2.1) are a useful guide as we plan our work, but virtually nothing we do fits neatly into any single strategy.

**Table 2.1. The Robert Wood Johnson Foundation
Communications Department Mission, *continued.***

5. Maintaining the quality and volume of the Foundation's proposal
   stream by
   • Stimulating interest among eligible organizations capable of taking
     actions consistent with the Foundation's mission
   • Providing potential applicants with information that is clear and
     precise about the Foundation's (i) intent, (ii) its interests and
     priorities, (iii) what it does not fund, and (iv) its application
     process
   • When appropriate, conducting a "call for proposals" process that
     creates a climate of receptivity and attracts highly qualified applicants
     who might otherwise never approach the Foundation.
6. Orchestrating two-way information flows with decision makers,
   opinion leaders, and other groups important to the Foundation's
   programmatic and philanthropic goals.
7. Ensuring the Foundation is appropriately accountable as the steward of
   private funds serving the public good. Techniques include:
   • Publishing an annual report, a quarterly publication focused on the
     work of our grantees, reports on the results of most programs, and an
     annual anthology of in-depth examinations of selected activities
   • Maintaining a website that includes all of the Foundation's
     publications and news releases and connections to grantee websites
   • Encouraging grantees to give appropriate notice of the Foundation's
     assistance in their publications, on their websites, and in contacts with
     news media and others
   • Maintaining effective relations with key news media
   • Ensuring a steady, two-way flow of useful information between the
     Foundation and decision makers and opinion leaders affecting health,
     health care, and the philanthropic community.

*Strategic communications is the managed process by which information
is produced and conveyed to achieve specific objectives vital to an organization's mission.

Everything we do is designed to advance multiple strategies,
although one is often dominant. A news release announcing a competitive grants program, for example, is primarily a way to let potential applicants know about our new funding interests (strategy #5),
but it also serves to make the Foundation more accountable (strategy
#7). And our website (www.rwjf.org) has become a key means for pur-
suing all of our strategies.

The website is also illustrative of our efforts to stay abreast of technological advances in communications and to incorporate them into the Foundation's armamentarium when they are sufficiently developed and effective. For example, in 1981 we first used teleconferencing, employing the facilities of public television stations to link grantees and local officials in 19 cities in launching our Program to Consolidate Health Services for High-Risk Young People. About that time, an initiative presenting the work of our grantees on commercial television was made possible through contractual arrangements with a health magazine show reaching 70 percent of the nation's homes. The Foundation's all-text "gopher" on the Internet was replaced in 1996 with a website, and a few years later we used similar technology to create an intranet site for Foundation staff and an extranet site linking the Foundation and its national program offices.

What gives life and substance to all of these words is people. Staff members in the Communications Department have varied experience and education. They come with skills including journalism, public relations, advertising, social marketing, public health and public administration, film and television production, policy analysis, publications design and production, institutional planning, and information science. They also bring knowledge of the health sector from their previous positions with university medical centers and hospitals, as journalists reporting health and health care, and with voluntary health associations, advocacy groups, government, and other foundations.

⎯⎯ Building Communications Into Programs

While examining the various activities and products of the Foundation's Communications Department, one should keep in mind the two contexts within which we work. The first is the seven strategies found in Table 2.1 in the previous section. These are the touchstones that give coherence to our work. The second is the uneven communications capacities of our grantees or their willingness to provide communications backup to the projects we support. For some grantees, such as an academic medical center, a Foundation-funded program may be only a small aspect of their overall work. We also cannot assume that grantees are as prepared to undertake the communications aspect of their projects as they are to run a clinic, conduct postdoctoral training, or carry out the other, substantive activities for which the grant was made. Moreover, the motivations of the Foundation and its grantees may differ. For example, the physicians directing HMO pediatric services using grant funds to apply innovative approaches for identifying children with asthma may view their challenge as one of integrating this innovation into their services and making it work; for the Foundation, though, this is a field test of the innovation, and sharing the experiences of this project with other HMOs throughout the country is crucial to its success.

To address issues such as these, the Foundation's communications effort begins in the earliest stage of grant making, during program design and proposal review within the Program Management Teams, or PMTs, the Foundation's basic organizational units. Six officers and an equal number of senior consultants in the Communications Department spearhead these efforts to identify ways in which communications might advance the objectives of the program under consideration. How, for example, can community coalitions maintain cohesion among their constituents and effectively influence public attitudes and opinions? Or how can grantees of research or demonstration programs reach decision makers? The PMTs then incorporate provisions for carrying out the relevant communications activities into the grant. Grant budget lines for communications have become the norm rather than the exception. They provide funds for communications staff and for activities ranging from websites to the publication and distribution of policy briefs, and from news conferences to time for project directors to write journal articles.

──── Technical Assistance and Training

Once programs are funded and under way, the Department's officers and consultants in the PMTs use technical assistance and training to enhance the effectiveness of the grantees' communications activities. We provide a steady stream of technical assistance and advice to our grantees—including supplementing grantee mailing lists; finding and selecting local communications consultants; and assisting with message development, priority setting, and the multitude of other elements that comprise effective communication. We do this work by phone, fax, and e-mail; through site visits; and by dispatching consultants with specialized skills.

We also contract with organizations conducting media training and sponsor a workshop series teaching representatives of approximately 135 grantees a year the basics of strategic communications and guiding them through the development of communications plans for their projects. In addition, Foundation communications staff members organize and participate in an annual two-and-a-half-day workshop with the extended family of major grantees' communications directors and key consultants. Some 90 professionals attended the 1999 session.

With between 2,000 and 2,500 programs open for business and receiving Foundation funds on any given day, budgetary tradeoffs dictate difficult choices in targeting technical assistance. We try to assist programs that can benefit most from this help, whose staffs are open to this work, and whose success would have the greatest impact in terms of health and health care. However, our decisions are the products of judgment, not science, and we make our share of mistakes.

Much of the assistance to grantees is facilitated by the national program mechanism pioneered by the Foundation in its earliest years to support multisite initiatives. Currently, 87 national program offices oversee 1,218 project sites and related activities. Twenty-one of these 87 have full-time communications staff members, and most of the others have consultants to assist them with their communications. By concentrating our technical assistance on these intermediary professionals—who then provide technical assistance to their far more numerous project sites—the Foundation's communications assistance is more of a wholesale, rather than a retail, operation. The diversity of the programs managed in this way testifies to the flexibility of the national program mechanism, including its embedded communications component—from Covering Kids, assisting efforts of all 50 states and the District of Columbia to enroll all eligible children in Medicaid and state child-health insurance programs, to Faith in Action, with more than 1,000 interfaith organizations of volunteers helping people with long-term health problems to remain in their homes; and from the Minority Medical Faculty Development Program, providing fellowships for minority physicians interested in academic medical careers and in fostering development of succeeding classes of minority physicians, to SmokeLess States, coalitions in 28 states and the District of Columbia working to reduce tobacco use through education, treatment, and policy initiatives.

It bears repeating, however, that technical assistance and training are costly and that a careful weighing of need, readiness, and anticipated outcome determines the degree of communications support for each program. Not surprisingly, most of our technical assistance involves helping grantees make their findings and lessons learned available to others. We do this to drive innovation and improvement by moving new knowledge and new ways of doing things into the mainstreams of practice and policy, and by opening new avenues of thinking and action.

While grantees have the primary responsibility for sharing their findings and experiences, in many circumstances this can be done more effectively and efficiently by combining the Foundation's resources with those of the grantee. For example, the Foundation collaborates with Henry Wechsler, of Harvard University, in planning, preparing for, and orchestrating national news conferences and scores of follow-up media appearances on his series of college binge drinking studies. Combining resources also makes particular sense when the task involves disseminating the experiences of multiple grantees, such as collaborating with staff members of community-based grantees around the country to provide advice and opportunities for the outreach components of the various PBS television series supported by the Foundation.

⸺ Communications as an Intervention

Over the years, too, we have come to see communications as an intervention that can be used to bring about change, particularly in encouraging attitudes, behaviors, and policies promoting good health—a concept that lies at the heart of our work combating substance abuse in the forms of tobacco, alcohol, and illicit drugs.

Today, Communications Department officers are responsible for overseeing and assisting grantees conducting major communications campaigns aimed at changing harmful behavior patterns. Two examples are the Partnership for a Drug-Free America and the National Center for Tobacco-Free Kids. The Partnership uses its talented staff, organizational experience, and high-level contacts in the advertising, marketing, and public relations communities to be a partner in the federal campaign to reduce the demand for illegal drugs among the nation's young people. This five-year, $1 billion federal initiative is the largest and most comprehensive public health campaign ever undertaken by the federal government.

The National Center for Tobacco-Free Kids has earned a reputation as a key national resource for media, policymakers, and public health organizations on issues regarding tobacco use by young people. Its staff, comprising top-notch communications, marketing, and policy professionals, has augmented and strengthened the skills of individuals and organizations working in state and local tobacco prevention. Center staff members also provide assistance to ensure that youth tobacco issues are front and center on the policy agenda.

Two other initiatives illustrate how communications as a primary intervention can address issues of health care, as distinct from behavioral health issues. The first is Last Acts, a nationwide campaign launched by the Communications Department in 1996. It is the Foundation's first initiative in what has subsequently become an extensive portfolio of grants to improve end-of-life care. More than 400 organizations have signed on as Partners, signifying their participation in raising awareness and taking steps in and through their own organizations to improve end-of-life care. They include most of the major associations of health professionals and institutions, important faith groups, the federal Department of Veteran Affairs, and the American Association of Retired Persons. This campaign—through the products of its task forces, its various meetings and conferences, the media coverage it generates, and its Partners' actions—is successfully building a base of public and professional support for improving end-of-life care. Three examples: (1) just before the trial of Dr. Jack Kevorkian in 1999, Last Acts' consultants provided journalists covering the trial with information about positive alternatives to suicide, which many of them incorporated into their coverage; (2) a workplace task force has developed a model employee benefits package for high-quality, comprehensive end-of-life care; and (3) Last Acts' definition of palliative care—known as "The Precepts"—offers guidance for patients, policy makers, and health providers for end-of-life care, and is now quoted in medical literature as the most up-to-date and accepted summarization. At this writing, in keeping with our tradition of doing our work through grantees, plans are being drawn to transfer management responsibility for Last Acts to an external organization, which would receive grant support for this work.

The other initiative was launched by the Communications Department in 1999 to build greater public awareness of the increasing number of people without health insurance, the accompanying tangle of problems they face, the tragic health consequences, and the proposed solutions to this vexing issue. Key elements of this effort include: (1) educating journalists about the issue of health coverage; (2) visiting key newspaper and magazine editorial boards to persuade them to write about the uninsured and on the specifics of proposed solutions; (3) encouraging and assisting people in communities across the country to write and place columns on the nation's op-ed pages; and (4) analyzing the quality of news coverage of this issue.

The campaign was kicked off by HealthCoverage 2000, a one-day conference held in January in Washington, D.C., attended by 425 journalists, policy makers and analysts, and national representatives of health-sector associations. Representatives of the eight cosponsoring organizations, led by Families USA and the Health Insurance Association of America, each presented a specific proposal for significantly decreasing the number of people without health care coverage in this country.[5] Humorously referred to as the "strange bedfellows conference" by some Washington insiders owing to the diversity of interests and points of view represented, this event sparked major attention in the media and among health care leaders, prompting the Foundation and the cosponsors to begin scheduling a series of similar, regional meetings for immediately after the November 2000 elections.

—— Working With News and Entertainment Media

Another priority of the Communications Department is improving media reporting on health and health care. The Foundation has supported such coverage on National Public Radio's "Morning Edition" and "All Things Considered" since 1986. More recently, we have begun funding the health desk on Public Radio International's "Market Place." In addition, we underwrite a competitive grants initiative through the Benton Foundation that supports health and health-care programming by local public radio stations.[6] WSKG Public Broadcasting, in Binghamton, New York, for example, used its grant to support a 19-county program of town meetings and conferences, special radio and television programming, a project website, and educational materials housed in the permanent reserve collections of 50 different libraries—all aimed at helping people understand their options for end-of-life care.

We have also long been supporters of relevant specials and series on national public television. The audience demographics of public radio and television make these media particularly attractive locations for calling attention to, and informing people about, important issues as well as innovations in health and health care. In the fall of 2000, for example, PBS is scheduled to broadcast ten hours of television programming with major funding from the Foundation for both production and extensive outreach to engage people across the country in relevant civic action. End-of-life issues are the focus of Bill Moyers's four-part series, *On Our Own Terms*, and Hedrick Smith's three-hour special, *How Good Is Our Health Care*, is to be preceded by a related, hour-long "Frontline" documentary he produced, *Dr. Solomon's Dilemma*, documenting the changes that market forces are making on a Harvard-affiliated Boston teaching hospital.

This aspect of our work has been reported in a chapter of the 1998-99 *Anthology*, but it's worth repeating that what drives our funding is broadcasting's role, which is "central to certain aspects of modern life:

- Setting the public and political agenda
- Describing the cultural context for decisions about the policy issues of the day
- Suggesting alternative visions for how some aspect of social and economic systems could work
- Giving an increasingly diverse society some common reference points (values, history, ideas)
- Serving as the primary source of news for large numbers of Americans
- Shaping people's perceptions of the 'other' in society."[7]

Mass and professional print media and the newer web-based news sites share these roles with broadcasting, which accounts for our interest in media generally. We round out our efforts to improve the quality entertainment media's depictions of the health and health care matters relevant to our program interests—showing the consequences, for example, of a character's substance abuse—by supporting organizations working with writers and producers seeking insight and information into that aspect of their craft. To improve health and health care reporting, our grant making has targeted organizations and institutions similarly helping journalists to improve the quality of print and broadcast news. Currently, for example, we fund a series of bimonthly briefings on relevant topics and issues for news professionals in New York with the Columbia University Graduate School of Journalism, in Washington with the Alliance for Health Reform, and in Chicago with the Northwestern University Medill School of Journalism.

All of the foregoing media efforts are separate and distinct from our work, and that of our grantees, to pitch specific stories to journalists, as well as to serve as information sources on topics central to our programs. Using time-honored public relations techniques to gain and improve coverage is a staple in our efforts to reach various publics with information important to improving health and health care.

⟶ A Few Words About 'Bad Press'

No organization of any size and reach that is active in a field like health care is immune from scrutiny and criticism, but, even so, The Robert Wood Johnson Foundation has had relatively few painful encounters with the media. The first such encounter, in the early 1970s, grew out of a New Brunswick political action group's attacks on Foundation grants to a local hospital. The grants were made for land acquisitions, and these acquisitions were displacing people who lived in rental properties that were to be razed to make way for expanded hospital and medical facilities. There were skirmishes in the local media—and the first-ever picketing of the Foundation—but perseverance eventually made it possible for the hospital to improve and expand its service to the community and the region by becoming a university teaching hospital with adjoining clinical facilities of the Robert Wood Johnson Medical School of the University of Medicine and Dentistry of New Jersey.

Across the country, the Foundation has occasionally come under fire from groups opposed to the development of school-based health care centers. It was tough going in Utah, and in Miami opponents attempted to rally support by a variety of means, including a plane flying over local beaches with a banner demanding that the Foundation "go home." Media coverage, as might be expected, was heavy as both sides sought to present their case to the public. The school centers were approved, and continue to this day with local funding and strong parental support.

Public debate involving the Foundation reached its most vigorous point in the last decade as a result of federal and state attempts to reform health care and expand health insurance coverage. We organized a series of community meetings so that people around the country could tell their stories and express their views, pro and con, to Hillary Clinton, who was then heading the Administration's efforts at reform. Because of this, and because so many of our grantees were involved in that Presidential initiative, hostile critics of the Foundation accused us of partisanship, and were widely quoted. We also made it possible for NBC News to produce and broadcast an ad-free prime-time special on reform issues by buying the commercial time. The critics added this to their charges of partisanship even though viewers, in two national surveys, found the show balanced and fair.

The headline of a national business magazine's opinion piece on our state-based grant making went over the top: "In Bed With the Devil." A couple of years later, the same magazine toned down its headline to "Trojan Horse Money," but the text was equally hostile among other things likening Foundation grants to bribes. Most of the truly one-sided accusatory articles, however, have appeared in relatively obscure newsletters published by partisan think tanks.

A Pennsylvania legislative hearing a few years ago, investigating foundation support of school health projects, included a day of testimony by a Kentucky lawyer who recycled accusations from the past and lambasted us mostly for allegations that had nothing to do with the supposed focus of the hearing. To see if there was any fire in these clouds of smoke, we commissioned a prominent Pennsylvania law firm to examine all allegations made involving our foundation. The investigating attorneys concluded that "the Subcommittee's conclusions about the Foundation and its grants to Pennsylvania agencies are unfounded," and backed up this finding with 36 pages of point-by-point refutation of the Subcommittee's own report.[8] An editorial in *The Philadelphia Inquirer*, commenting on the hearings, put it more colorfully by calling on the Subcommittee chairman to "focus his tax-payer-funded investigative efforts on something a bit more sensible. UFOs in the school cafeteria?"[9]

A good communications staff can help ensure that an organization's points of view aren't overlooked in media accounts of conflict—and that an organization doesn't shoot itself in the foot by being lured into unnecessary and futile public debate. But the most important point is that in our free and open society, foundations, like everyone else, have to be willing to take public criticism, and even public attack, if they want to use their funds effectively to help solve important social problems. Steven Schroeder, our president, told a *Wall Street Journal* reporter, "To avoid controversy means doing things that are so bland that they aren't important. We're going to get our share of potshots. It's a risk that we have to take."[10]

⎯⎯ Making Connections—A New Approach to Technical Assistance

Helping to connect grantees with the media and prepare them for interviews is, as noted earlier, a time-honored approach to getting the word out in keeping with our technical assistance and dissemination strategies. A new initiative known as Connect extends this approach from media to include the grantees' local congressional delegations and their staffs. It offers broad benefits all around.

Grantees gain the attention of people who can open doors for them in their communities, states, and even nationally. The members of Congress get to meet interesting constituents with on-the-ground, back-home expertise and experience dealing with a variety of health and health care issues and challenges. In Maryland, a Congressman met with representatives of an interfaith caregivers project in his district and pitched in to help them identify potential clients who might use the shopping, housekeeping, transportation, and other services offered by the project's volunteers. Members of his staff have since worked with the project to provide letters of support for new funding requests, organize in-kind donations from local businesses, and identify new opportunities for media coverage. A California Congressman visiting a clinic in his district funded by the Foundation's Reach Out program learned that most of the patients cared for by the clinic's volunteer physicians were employed by small businesses unable to afford health insurance for their workers. He volunteered to help the clinic raise funds to cover its administrative expenses from the local business community. And a Senator from the Southwest was so affected by the work of a program battling substance abuse in one of his state's small communities that he returned and chaired a Senate subcommittee hearing there on substance abuse problems along the U.S.-Mexican border. The list of such stories is long and continues to grow.

The Foundation and philanthropy in general also benefit. Ours is an "industry" regulated by Congress, and the Connect initiative serves to enhance our accountability. It gives members of Congress and their staffs the opportunity to talk with Foundation staff members arranging the visits and to gain insight into how foundations work and the special role that they play in American life. We invite local reporters and correspondents to the visits; and everyone involved benefits from the resulting coverage, including the media, which thrive on interesting stories. If the grantees also have support from local foundations, we include their representatives in the visits and the publicity, thereby sharing the benefits even more widely.

∼ Contributing to the Learning Environment

One of the Foundation's current objectives is to create an environment that fosters building on experience, our own as well as the accumulated knowledge and experiences of others. The Communications Department's contributions to this learning environment—in keeping with our strategy to share information from our work and that of our grantees—are the Foundation's *Annual Report*; our quarterly news publication *Advances*; the Foundation's website (www.rwjf.org); the Foundation's Information Center; and two projects I oversee jointly with the Foundation's vice president for research and evaluation, my department's Grant Results Reporting Unit and the annual publication *To Improve Health and Health Care: The Robert Wood Johnson Foundation Anthology*.

The **Annual Report** serves a blend of purposes. It is a historical record that, by virtue of its distribution to 22,000 individuals on our mailing list and to countless others through posting on our website, serves our commitment to make the Foundation accountable and accessible. It offers the why, the whom, and for what purposes we made our grant and contract investments; our audited financial statements; selected excerpts from the bibliography of information materials produced with Foundation support; the names of trustees, staff, and others, including national program directors, responsible for the Foundation and its programs; guidance on applying for grants; and a biographical sketch and tribute to Robert Wood Johnson, whose vision and generosity created and put the Foundation into motion. The *Annual Report*'s final ingredient is the President's statement, a platform each of our three presidents—David E. Rogers, Leighton E. Cluff, and Steven A. Schroeder—has used to add intellectual and moral context to our work and mission. Each has penned his own essays, and the quality of the thinking and writing in this now-substantial body of work is as much a tribute to the trustees who have selected our presidents as it is to the authors themselves. One man's opinion, but I believe both groups have set extraordinarily high standards for their successors.

Advances, focusing principally on the work of our grantees (and not our staff), is now mailed to between 40,000 and 60,000 people (we add special groups to the core list depending on featured topics). In readership studies we do every three or four years, *Advances* consistently draws good reviews; invariably, there is a surge of requests for other Robert Wood Johnson Foundation publications after they have been featured in *Advances;* and each month we receive approximately 120 requests from individuals to be added to the *Advances* mailing list, which more than offsets attrition.

The **Foundation's website** offers a near-limitless collection of news and archived information about the Foundation and its grant-assisted projects, including the text and graphics of all the print materials we have produced since 1996 and some basic materials from before that. At this writing, the content is the equivalent of 46,000 pages of text, growing at the rate of 276 pages weekly, and the site is receiving more than 16,000 visits per week, up more than 50 percent from the prior year. Handling information on this scale is a formidable and costly enterprise. We're proud of what we have achieved, but the site is still a long way from where we want it to be. Critics tell us that it should be more user friendly. Navigation is daunting; there is too much foundation and academic jargon; and too often the contexts and perspectives are the Foundation's rather than the public's—"Too much inside baseball," one critic put it. We continue to make improvements, and we've learned that in the fast-moving worlds of technology and the health sector, a website such as ours will always be a work in progress. Nonetheless, in 1998, e-mail messages via our website surpassed U.S. mail as the means by which we receive most requests for Foundation publications. And the transition from a passive bulletin board and file cabinet of information to a place of interactivity and community building began just over a year ago with creation of a joined-at-the-hip website for the Last Acts program as a virtual section of the Foundation's website.

The *Anthology*, now in its fourth volume, features case studies and analyses providing in-depth looks into the Foundation's own processes and the programs that it funds. The book is mailed each year without charge to more than 12,000 individuals with key roles in the philanthropic and health sectors, including all current grantees, and then marketed and sold by the publisher, Jossey-Bass. All the volumes are also posted on our website.

The staff of four in our **Grant Results Reporting Unit** supervises the work of almost 70 freelance writers and editors preparing accounts, from one to sixty pages, on grantee accomplishments with Foundation funds. To date, the unit has produced summaries and analyses of projects and programs encompassing more than 700 grants, all posted to our website. This work is now hitting its stride, and reports encompassing another 500 grants are in production. This record of what has been accomplished with the Foundation's funds is being mined for lessons, and is already sparking change internally. The reports also offer potential grant applicants insight into our funding interests and strategies, and promise to become a rich source of data and information for other grant makers and for historians, health service researchers, and other scholars.

The **Information Center** undergirds all of the Department's activities, and much of the Foundation's program work as well. In morphing from library to Information Center, this unit has undergone an electronic-age revitalization. The web and other electronic services now lead print materials by a 2:1 margin as sources used by Center staff in filling the 100 or so staff information requests processed monthly. Center staff members also conduct specific electronic searches periodically to inform Foundation officers of new developments in their fields. And Foundation staff members have access, via their desktop computers, to the Information Center's card catalog, Lexis-Nexis, updated lists of work-relevant websites, and a variety of other electronic databases. But print lives on: in addition to a book collection of more than 3,000 volumes, the Center circulates 313 periodicals and processes 150 requests monthly for books and journal articles via an interlibrary loan system.

⁓ The Future of Foundation Communications

Although foundations have resisted using communications, powerful forces for change are underway that make communication vital to their operations. These forces are moving foundations into more active, broader public engagement—to build funding and issue alliances on behalf of their own program interests, to support their own role in the modern world, and to enable them to respond effectively to their grantees' needs—and they are stocking communications toolkits essential for this work. The driving forces include:

- The dynamics of our republic and its evolved capitalist economy, with a suspicion of élites as a recurring thread in its social fabric, and with an increasingly diverse population

- The idea that foundations ought to be investors in innovation and social capital rather than dispensers of charity, attacking root problems rather than ameliorating symptoms

- The ascendancy of three propositions: (1) that while foundation funds are private, they are to be used for the public good; (2) that foundations should therefore be publicly accountable for what they do; and (3) that funds put into foundations by their donors represent "tax expenditures" because some large share of them would otherwise have become tax revenues

- Legislation and public policy that makes organized philanthropy, especially foundations, answerable to and regulated by federal and state government

- The emergence of information coupled with new communications technologies as social, political, and economic drivers

- The shrinking value of foundations' financial assets relative to the magnitude and complexity of the problems they address, plus the emergence of the federal government and multilateral entities as even greater forces within foundations' domains of action.

That last point contains the seeds of what I believe are the most powerful forces propelling private foundations to embrace *strategic* communications. Go back to the halcyon years of foundations—the 1920s and the next several decades—a historical period I studied and came to appreciate when I was a program officer at the Commonwealth Fund and later when I served as vice president for communications at the Rockefeller Foundation. This was the period when the first of our country's foundations came to prominence and gained renown for the social change they sparked. Modern medical education, the entire field of public health, the elimination of hookworm in the South, the Green Revolution—these are hoary stories that old Rockefeller Foundation coots like me tell our grandchildren and foundation officers new to the field. In those good old days, a Rockefeller Foundation could single-handedly take on and defeat a world-class problem. Why didn't these golden years continue into the present?

As my examples imply, the most powerful way that foundations can spark social change is to use their money to fund the creation of new institutions or fundamental change in existing institutions. The *cJP*

Table 2.2.   Operating Budgets (in millions of dollars).

	1930	1999
Harvard Medical School	$ 1	$ 286
Johns Hopkins University	3	1,699
Children's Hospital of Philadelphia	0.2	716
Federal Research and Development (excluding census)	43	75,351
Rockefeller Foundation Grants	15	175

Sources for institutional funding are from personal communications with the institutions and for the federal government are from the National Science Foundation, Division of Science Resources Studies, *Federal Funds for Research and Development: Fiscal years 1998, 1999, and 2000*, NSF 00-317, Project Officer, Ronald L. Meeks (Arlington, Virginia 2000), and A. H. Dupree, *Science in the Federal Government* (Baltimore, Maryland: Johns Hopkins University Press, 1986), page 331.

first column in Table 2.2 is the 1930 operating budget of a number of important American institutions and programs, together with the federal government's overall research and development budget and the total of Rockefeller Foundation grants.

It's clear that in 1930 the Rockefeller Foundation had the financial means to exercise the strategy of building and reshaping institutions to a fare-thee-well. But by 1995, column two, the proportion of Rockefeller funds to the other budgets had become altogether different, and it had been so for some time. No longer was the Rockefeller Foundation a powerhouse for social change using the strategy of institutional creation and change. Nor was, or is, any other foundation today.[11] An amount of money equal to The Robert Wood Johnson Foundation's annual grant making comes and goes in this country's current trillion-dollar-a-year health expenditures between midnight, January 1, and dawn of that first day. The strategies for social change we must use today—research and policy analysis, training, demonstrations, advocacy, as well as coalition building and attempts to leverage the actions of others—are all heavily dependent on effective communications. So, too, are the funding and grantee coalitions that are ubiquitous today. Further, compared with those earlier years, our country is almost awash with foundations, public charities, and government agencies, all competing for space and time in the proliferating channels and numbing volume of public and private communication—additional drivers for the use of strategic communications.

There are signs that all these factors and trends are turning the foundation world toward the acceptance of strategic communications as a tool for advancing program objectives, whether they be in health and health care or in the arts, education, environmental sciences, or any of the myriad other fields in which foundations labor. Foundation annual and special reports, grant guidelines, newsletters, and magazines fill office in-boxes. Foundation-sponsored PBS programs and NPR reportage have become commonplace. Foundations and their grantees sponsor town meetings, community and statewide coalition building, and grassroots organizing across the country on everything from the future of Social Security to the protection of children from substance abuse. Foundations by the dozen design, post, and link up their own websites.

Within the field, regional associations of grant makers are busy helping their member foundations, small as well as large, learn more about communications, while both the Council on Foundations and Independent Sector have launched large-scale communications efforts. When the Council held its 50th annual conference, in 1999, the theme was—you guessed it—communications. And the Communications Network, which began 21 years ago as an informal gathering of foundation communications officers, has grown into a nonprofit organization whose mission is to help foundation trustees, CEOs and program officers, as well as communications officers, sharpen their communications thinking and skills.

Only slowly, however, are foundations learning to be strategic. This means, in bare-bones terms: (1) having a vision for how some segment of the world might be better; (2) mapping the field in terms of forces bearing on the vision; (3) choosing and pursuing one or more specific objectives that seem doable and whose potential for moving the chosen segment of the world toward the vision seems greater than alternative objectives; and (4) harnessing the power of communications to support this work.

—— Communications and the Road Ahead

The greatest void in our communications realm is knowledge of its effectiveness. We have included evaluations in specific communications efforts with varying degrees of success. We have print, radio, and television "clippings" from news conferences, survey results from periodic polls and readership studies, and a variety of other such indices, but almost never do we know with much certainty the degree to which our efforts have sparked change. Partly, this is because of the smallness of what we do compared to the vastness of information flows in health and health care. Partly, because of the difficulty of linking cause and effect in this complex, crowded domain. And partly because information is but one of the factors influencing change.

The evaluative tools we have for measuring effectiveness are also relatively crude, as is our understanding of how to use them effectively. For example, as described in the previously cited 1998-99 *Anthology* chapter on our radio and television grants, two separate measurements of audience effect by the 1994 NBC special on health care reform—evaluations designed and conducted by highly respected academic researchers—produced conflicting findings.[11]

The difficulty in measuring the effectiveness of communications is just one part of the larger difficulty in measuring the effectiveness of all philanthropic work whose intended outcome is social change. For us, hope for improvement lies in an effort of the Foundation's staff, still under way at this writing, to define measurable outcomes indicating progress toward program goals. These outcome targets will facilitate our developing similarly measurable, intermediate outcomes for our related and supporting communications work. Hope also lies in efforts just begun to incorporate more rigorously the thinking and the processes of social marketing in the Foundation's work. This will bring to bear the marketing techniques of audience research, segmentation, and analysis; exchange strategies; and information and communications targeting designed to shape perspectives and motivate action—all designed to produce substantially improved health and health care outcomes.

In addition, plans to continue increasing our use of Internet and web technologies may play a role in helping us to gauge the effectiveness of our communications. These technologies—besides offering relatively inexpensive, swift means to give people access to vast amounts of information—make possible heretofore impossible interactivity between the Foundation and its key publics. Out of this interactivity could come new insights into how information is used, and the effects of using it.

As one who is fast approaching retirement, I am optimistic that these anticipated efforts will materialize and go forward as planned, but I am mindful, too, of uncertainty. As that great American philosopher Yogi Berra once observed, "The future ain't what it used to be."[13]

Notes

1. Credit for the Foundation's communications work is properly shared with those who have contributed so much to its development. Three individuals played key roles in the formative years: William E. Walch, Andrew Burness, and Victoria D. Weisfeld. Currently, in addition to Weisfeld, nine other officers have raised communications to its present level: Joan K. Hollendonner, Joseph F. Marx, Stuart M. Schear, Paul A. Tarini, Ann E. Searight, Marian E. Bass, Hinda Greenberg, and Molly McKaughan. I also want to acknowledge the valued contributions of a good friend who was both my successor and predecessor, Thomas P. Gore, who served as the Foundation's vice president for communications from 1987 until 1993. Finally, a special note of thanks to Linda Bernstein Jasper for her assistance with this manuscript.

2. D. E. Rogers. "The President's Statement." *The Robert Wood Johnson Foundation Annual Report 1972*. Princeton, N.J.: The Robert Wood Johnson Foundation, 1972, p. 17.

3. D. E. Rogers. "The President's Statement." *The Robert Wood Johnson Foundation Annual Report 1974*. Princeton, N.J.: The Robert Wood Johnson Foundation, 1975, p. 14.

4. S. A. Schroeder, "Reflections on the Challenges of Philanthropy." *Health Affairs*, 1998, *17*, 209–216.

5. The other six organizations were the American Hospital Association, American Medical Association, American Nurses Association, Catholic Health Association of the United States, Service Employees International Union, and U.S. Chamber of Commerce.

6. This is discussed in D. Diehl, "Sound Partners for Community Health," in this year's *Anthology*.

7. V. D. Weisfeld. "The Foundation's Radio and Television Grants, 1987–1997." In S. L. Isaacs and J. R. Knickman, (eds.), *To Improve Health and Health Care 1998–1999: The Robert Wood Johnson Anthology*. San Francisco: Jossey-Bass, 1998, pp. 187–212.

8. R. S. Goldman and D. F. Abernathy. Final Report of the Select Subcommittee on House Resolution 37 of the Committee on Education of the Pennsylvania House of Representatives Dated November 19, 1996. Report to the Robert Wood Johnson Foundation, 14 July 1997.

9. "A Princeton Plot?" *The Philadelphia Inquirer*, 4 December 1995, A14.

10. G. Anders. "Foundation Is Accused of Playing Politics With Grants." *Wall Street Journal*, 26 April, 1994.

11. While a few of the largest foundations at this writing do have sufficient funds to pursue a strategy of institution building and change on a scale equal to that of the halcyon years, they would have to narrow the focus of

their grant making to a degree that seems highly unlikely, except, perhaps, in the case of The Bill and Melinda Gates Foundation.

12. See note 6, page 203.
13. Y. Berra, *The Yogi Book: I Really Didn't Say Everything I Said!* New York: Workman Publishers, 1998, pp. 118–119.

Programs

CHAPTER THREE

—∿— Children's Health Initiatives

Sharon Begley and Ruby P. Hearn

Editors' Introduction

Although improving the health of children has never been an explicit goal of The Robert Wood Johnson Foundation, its investments in the area have been substantial. In 1999, for example, slightly more than a third of the dollars awarded by the Foundation supported efforts to improve children's health. Given the scale of the Foundation's efforts, it is not surprising that each of the first three volumes of the *Anthology* included chapters examining specific children's health programs.

In this fourth volume of the *Anthology*, Sharon Begley, a senior editor at *Newsweek*, and Ruby Hearn, a senior vice president who has been an active advocate for children's concerns during more than a quarter-century at The Robert Wood Johnson Foundation, have undertaken a comprehensive look at the approaches the Foundation has adopted, and the programs it has supported, to improve children's health and well-being. They begin with some of the Foundation's earliest grants in the 1970s and take us through its latest investments.

Why the long-lived commitment to children? For some, the reasons are economic: investments in children's health can have enduring payoffs, enabling the young to become productive and healthy citizens in the future. For others, it is a matter of fairness: while children as a whole tend to be healthier than people in other age groups, children of minorities and lower-income families and those who live in rural areas and urban slums suffer disproportionately and have limited access to health care services. For many, it is a matter of morality: most of us would find it unconscionable to live in a society that scrimps on the care of its young people and turns the other way when children experience problems that could be avoided with new approaches to care and services.

This chapter examines the wide range of approaches employed by the Foundation—research, demonstrations, coalition building, communications, and financing strategies—to improve the health of children from newborns to adolescents. It shows how the Foundation's strategies have evolved in response to the changing social and political environment. And it offers observations on approaches to improving children's health based on more than a quarter-century of experience.

Since 1972, when The Robert Wood Johnson Foundation was established, it has awarded more than 2,000 grants, totaling over $860 million, to improve children's health and health care. That's a lot of grants and a lot of history.

From the beginning, grants in the field of children's health have been shaped by the Foundation's overall mission—to improve the health and health care of *all* Americans, young and old. Since the Foundation has never had an explicit goal of improving children's health, its children's health programs have generally followed its overall priorities. In the early years, that meant improving access to medical services. In the 1980s, improving the care of people with chronic illnesses began to receive the Foundation's attention. In 1991, the Foundation adopted three explicit goals: increasing access to care, reducing the harm caused by substance abuse, and improving chronic care services. As it happens, each of these is particularly relevant for children. In 1998, some 11.1 million children had no health insurance coverage, compared with 9.6 million in 1993. Many chronic illnesses have their antecedents in childhood. And among the many risk factors for substance abuse are the economic, social, and psychological forces that shape an individual's early years.

Children's Health and the Foundation's Priorities
Improving Access to Care

Early Childhood Programs

One of the most serious problems facing America's children in the 1970s was the unacceptably high infant mortality rate. As one of its earliest efforts in children's health, the Foundation chose a program to reduce deaths of newborns. The 1960s and 1970s saw the emergence of technologies (including those to stabilize a premature baby's respiration and control body temperature) that promised to do just that. The Foundation funded the Regionalized Perinatal Care Program (1975 to 1982), which organized hospitals in eight areas of the country into regional networks to make perinatal technology available to more women and their at-risk babies.[1] (Perinatal applies to the period shortly before and after birth.) The regionalization of perinatal services throughout the country—including those funded by The Robert Wood Johnson Foundation—contributed to a reduction in the nation's infant mortality rate from 18.5 deaths per 1,000 live births in 1972 to 7.2 deaths per 1,000 in 1997.

The next logical step was to bring the benefits of perinatal regionalization into the most isolated rural communities: thus was born the Rural Infant Care Program (1979 to 1985), which helped states organize collaborations between medical schools and public health departments to offer outpost clinics for underserved women and children. But would babies survive their infancy only to suffer later from developmental disabilities? To find out, the Foundation funded a study of the long-term development of low-birthweight babies. It found that these children were at an increased risk of cognitive and developmental problems by the time they reached 8 to 10 years of age.[2]

To improve the prospects for low-birthweight babies, the Foundation funded a large randomized clinical trial called the Infant Health and Development Program (1982 to 1991 and 1992 to 1994). This program provided the most promising interventions then available, such as home visits and infant day care with a defined curriculum, to low-birthweight babies. It then compared their health and development with low-birthweight babies who received only standard medical services. The evaluators found some differences in cognitive and developmental functions, though not enough to justify the high cost of the interventions. They also found that children could receive care in a communal setting without increasing the risk of infection.

Concurrent with these efforts was a trial that tested a different approach to improving the prospects of high-risk children. In 1979, the Foundation joined other institutions[3] in funding Dr. David Olds's plan to establish a program of home visits by registered nurses to about 400 unmarried, low-income pregnant women—most of whom were teenagers—in Elmira, a semirural town in upstate New York. The nurses provided prenatal care in-home visits every other week, and offered counseling on nutrition, avoiding smoking, parenting skills, and crisis management. They were available by phone at night and on weekends, and typically worked with the mothers for two years after the baby's birth. Unlike the Infant Health and Development Program, which provided services after babies were born, the visits by nurses began while women were still pregnant, in the expectation that better prenatal care would reduce the number of low-birthweight babies. In addition to providing prenatal care, the nurses encouraged women to stop smoking or using drugs; educated families about how to improve the baby's health; and, perhaps most important, helped the women become economically self-sufficient by getting them to plan subsequent pregnancies, continue their education, and find a job.

Follow-up studies—the children with whom Olds began the program in Elmira have been studied for more than 15 years—have found striking differences between children in the program and a control group. The program group experienced 79 percent fewer reports of child abuse and neglect, 44 percent less incidence of alcohol and drug use by the kids, and 54 percent lower frequency of arrests by age 15.[4] A RAND study concluded that for every dollar invested in visiting the at-risk women and their children, society reaped $4 in benefits.[5] "The differences arose, we think, not only from helping the mothers be more competent parents but also from helping them make better decisions about what kind of lives they wanted and what kind of men they wanted in their lives," says Olds, now a professor of pediatrics and nursing at the University of Colorado Health Sciences Center and director of the Kempe Prevention Research Center for Family and Child Health. "One woman told the nurse, 'I don't want to hang out with Tony anymore—he'll be a bad influence on the baby.' Through the continuing nurses' visits, the women developed a vision of what their life could be, and we think that is directly due to their involvement with the nurse." To test whether the approach would achieve the same results in a different setting, Olds repeated the program in 1987 in Memphis, Tennessee. Providing services to 1,100 families, the program had similar positive results. The Robert Wood Johnson Foundation is now supporting the replication of Olds's work by funding the development of technical resource centers across the country.

School-Based Health Programs

A different approach to improving access to health care for children and adolescents is bringing services to the place where young people spend most of their time—the school. The Foundation has supported school-based health services almost continuously since the 1970s.[6] The School Health Services Program (1977 to 1984) tested the benefits of providing a nurse practitioner to elementary schools. In 1986, the Foundation launched the School-Based Adolescent Health Care

Program. With grants of up to $600,000 for each location, the program established health centers in 24 high schools in 14 cities, including Detroit, Los Angeles, Miami, New Orleans, New York, San Fernando, and San Jose. To engage the communities at an early stage, the Foundation required that each center be planned in consultation with parents, school officials, health and welfare departments, and the business community, and that each clinic cooperate with the school nurses, counselors, and other staff members. Furthermore, each clinic had to work with a community advisory board that would both raise funds to support the clinic during the six years of the Foundation's grant and to keep it running after the grant expired.

By many measures, the school-based clinics seemed to be just what the doctor ordered. Despite concerns from the Catholic Church and some parents about the reproductive health services that the clinics made available, participation was high: 70 percent of the kids at the 24 schools got parental permission to use the facilities, and about 70 percent of those (half of the students) actually availed themselves of one service or another. The school-based clinics were particularly important in providing mental health services to students. Even though the clinics were able to provide many medical services to students, a 1993 evaluation found that they did not have a significant impact on two areas of particular concern: teenage pregnancy and drug use. In some schools, these issues were not even addressed. Where they were, whatever intervention was offered to head off those problems was apparently too little and too late.

Moreover, funding problems loomed, for neither Medicaid nor other insurers reimbursed the clinics for many of the preventive or mental health services they offered. The biggest blow came with the rise of managed care. Many Medicaid managed-care plans, which states were adopting because of the cost savings they promised, balked at designating the school clinics as eligible providers. Many health maintenance organizations and other managed-care plans feared that the clinics would not be able to provide all the health services the children needed. Partly as a result of these factors, the number of school-based clinics has stalled out at roughly 1,200—out of a total of 88,000 public schools in the country.[7] The Foundation's current school-based health program, Making the Grade (1992 to 2001), directly addresses the financing issues. It supports efforts in nine states to find mechanisms to improve the financing of school-based services. Most states in the program are trying to facilitate negotiations between school-based health centers and Medicaid managed care plans.

Insurance Coverage

Providing health services—through perinatal networks, in schools, or wherever—is one way of improving children's access to care; another way is offering insurance coverage to children.[8] The Healthy Kids Replication Program (1996 to 2001) took one approach to enrolling children in health insurance, helping states emulate a Florida program in which a school district is used as an insurance risk pool, thereby making thousands of kids eligible for group insurance. (Federal, state, and family funds are pooled to pay the premiums.)

The Covering Kids Program (1997 to 2002) takes a different approach. It seeks to identify uninsured children who are eligible for Medicaid or other state health insurance programs. Initially, the program contained funds to support programs in 15 states. However, shortly after the trustees approved the program in 1997, Congress authorized $24 billion over five years for a State Children's Health Insurance Program, or CHIP, with a goal of enrolling five million low-income children in Medicaid or state health insurance programs. With the passage of CHIP, The Robert Wood Johnson Foundation expanded Covering Kids to cover all 50 states and the District of Columbia. The two approaches complement each other: federal and state funds are used primarily to buy care for eligible children; the Foundation's funds are used largely to find them. CHIP, however, has fallen far short of its target; in 1999, President Clinton called it "simply inexcusable that we're sitting here, and have been, with the money for two years to provide health insurance to five million kids, and 80 percent of them are still uninsured." Early in 2000, the Foundation intensified its efforts, authorizing a $26 million, 3-year effort to enhance the public's understanding of why covering children is so important and to reach out to eligible children and their families.

Immunizations

One long-standing challenge has been getting children vaccinated at the appropriate time. This problem is due, in part, to the lack of any systematic way of knowing which children have been immunized and when their next shot is due. With the rise in managed care turning the doctor-patient relationship into a version of musical chairs, children's vaccination records often get lost in the shuffle, and doctors overestimate the percentage of their patients who are up-to-date on their shots by 40 percent.[9] A logical approach is to create immunization registries for children. The All Kids Count Program (1992 to 1997 and 1998 to 2002) seeks to improve the rate of childhood immunization by creating a database that records all the vaccinations a child receives and provides reminders when another is due.[10] Even as the Foundation has supported the effort to develop registries, a small backlash against immunizations has arisen. This led the Foundation to fund, in 2000, a new program of the American Society of Infectious Diseases to help patients and providers understand the risks and the benefits of vaccinations.

Chronic Care

In the late 1980s, when the Foundation began to address certain chronic illnesses and after 1991 when improving chronic care became a Foundation goal, programs for children followed. The Mental Health Services Program for Youth (1988 to 1997) reorganized available funding for children with severe mental illness so that, instead of being institutionalized, they could receive community-based care or home-based care.[11] It placed the children and their parents at the center of a system of services involving health care, mental health care, education, child welfare and, when needed, juvenile justice. The evaluators found that the eight sites in the program expanded the range and the flexibility of services available to children, but "fell short of fully developed systems of care."[12]

One of the most ambitious attempts to help children with chronic illnesses was a demonstration project called the Child Health Initiative. (More formally, it was named Improving Child Health Services: Removing Categorical Barriers to Care—1990 to 1997.) It grew out of the recognition that the services and interventions that children need are often compartmentalized in many different programs administered by an alphabet soup of federal, state, and local agencies. By 1994, there were nearly 500 federal programs funding children's services in narrowly defined categories.[13] Each service has a different funding source, different eligibility requirements, and different application procedures—not exactly what poor families need. The idea of the Child Health Initiative was to pool existing funds that a family or a child was eligible for and use them where they were most needed. This was called decategorizing funds.

More recently, since asthma is the most prevalent chronic illness among children, the Foundation is supporting Allies Against Asthma

(1998 to 2003), a program designed by the federal Centers for Disease Control and Prevention to help communities reduce allergens by teaching families how to rid a home of, say, dust mites.

Substance Abuse

When the Foundation began to address the harm caused by substance abuse in the late-1980s, the children's health programs took up the cause. The Fighting Back Program (1988 to 2003) takes a community approach to reducing the demand for tobacco, alcohol, and illegal drugs. Although Fighting Back supports community coalitions to decrease substance abuse among people of all ages, in practice it has focused largely on children. In Newark, New Jersey, for example, the grantee uses the program's funds to station police officers in drug-ridden public housing projects with the simple goal of getting kids to school safely and without encountering dealers. A different approach has been taken by the Free to Grow Program (1992 to 2005) which works with Head Start—the nation's largest publicly funded early childhood development program—to strengthen families and communities in their efforts to prevent substance abuse. In Puerto Rico, for instance, the Head Start program went beyond its usual mandate of getting preschoolers ready to learn, and paired troubled families with godparent families that helped the former find jobs and counseling.

To capitalize on the stature of athletes in their communities, the Foundation is supporting the Jacksonville Jaguars Honor Rows Program (1995 to 2001). The team offers free home-game tickets to disadvantaged kids who sign pledges to avoid tobacco, alcohol, and illegal drugs, successfully do so, and attain certain academic, behavior, and public service goals. Recognizing that many people get hooked on tobacco as teenagers, the foundation joined with 20 other organizations in the mid-1990s to develop a Campaign for Tobacco-Free Kids. This led to the establishment of the National Center for Tobacco-Free Kids (1996 to 2004), which focuses on countering the tobacco industry's youth-oriented advertising with an antismoking campaign. The Smoke-Free Families Program (1993 to 2003) funds projects aimed at preventing the birth of low-birthweight babies by helping pregnant women kick the nicotine habit. The idea is that expecting a baby—when women are the most concerned about the harm that tobacco might do to their child—gives women an extra incentive to quit.

ঞৌ৸

Table 3.1.   National Programs on Children's Health of
The Robert Wood Johnson Foundation.

Name	Years	Funding Amount*
Regionalized Perinatal Care Program	1975–1983	$21,395,966
School Health Services Program	1977–1984	5,763,745
Rural Infant Care Program	1979–1985	8,338,645
Infant Health and Development Program	1982–1991	33,522,368
Family Friends: A Program to Enable Older Volunteers to Assist Disabled Children and Their Families	1985–1991	5,391,264
School-Based Adolescent Health Care Program	1986–1993	18,164,465
Healthy Futures: A Program to Improve Maternal and Infant Care in the South	1987–1994	9,408,860
Fighting Back: Community Initiatives to Reduce Demand for Illegal Drugs and Alcohol	1988–2003	72,600,000
Mental Health Services Program for Youth	1988–1997	24,164,077
Improving Child Health Services: Removing Categorical Barriers to Care	1990–1997	7,283,136
All Kids Count: Establishing Immunization Monitoring and Follow-up Systems	1991–2000	20,550,000
Free to Grow: Head Start Partnerships to Promote Substance-Free Communities	1992–2005	13,400,000
Infant Health and Development Program Replication	1992–1994	1,500,000
Making the Grade: State and Local Partnerships to Establish School-Based Health Centers	1992–2001	16,600,000
Mental Health Services Program for Youth Replication	1993–1997	1,001,549
Smoke-Free Families: Innovations to Stop Smoking During and Beyond Pregnancy	1993–2003	20,450,000
Dissemination of a Model Injury Prevention Program for Children and Adolescents (Injury Free Coalition for Kids)	1994–2001	4,300,648

⤜⤛

Table 3.1. National Programs on Children's Health of
The Robert Wood Johnson Foundation, *continued.*

Name	Years	Funding Amount*
Urban Health Initiative: Working to Ensure the Health and Safety of Children	1995–2002	34,000,000
Healthy Kids Replication Program	1996–2001	3,000,000
National Center for Tobacco-Free Kids	1996–2004	70,000,000
Covering Kids: A National Health Access Initiative for Low-Income, Uninsured Children	1997–2002	47,000,000
The Collaborative Center for Child Health And Development	1999–2001	9,000,000
Nurse Home-Visiting Program for First-Time, Low-Income Mothers and Their Newborns	1999–2002	10,000,000

* For closed programs, the funding amount is total spending including planning, evaluation, technical assistance, and other expenses. For active programs, the funding amount is the current authorization for implementation.

—— Evolution of the Foundation's Approaches to Improving Children's Health

Beyond evolving to fit within the Foundation's priorities, the Foundation's children's health programs have changed over the years to meet the shifting environment of social policy. In the process of this evolution, a number of insights have emerged about developing programs to improve children's health.

From Demonstration Programs to Large Programs That Engage the Community

In the 1970s, the Foundation developed the model of testing different approaches to solving problems through demonstration programs carried out at different locations around the country. These controlled studies were carefully evaluated in the expectation that the federal government would pick up and expand those approaches that appeared successful. That model worked in the case of AIDS patients, for instance. When the program demonstrated that this model of care worked beyond San Francisco, where it began, it paved the way for the Ryan White Act, which funded such care. That was the traditional Robert Wood Johnson Foundation model.

By the late 1980s, however, it was clear that this "build it and they will come" (or, at least, fund it) approach would no longer fly. Even a program shown by follow-up evaluation to have worked will not necessarily be scaled up or expanded on that basis alone. It rarely happens "that facts determined by scientific method . . . lead to policy change," a 1992 evaluation of the Foundation's maternal and child health programs warned.[14] Take school-based health care. As noted earlier, the programs have reached only 1,200 of 88,000 elementary and secondary schools in the country. For kids with access to one of those 1,200 schools, of course, the clinics are as welcome as a hot shower after a gritty soccer practice: the staff treats sore throats before they bloom into full-scale strep infections, oversees asthma medication before the wheezing child lands in the emergency room, and even runs interference with teachers for troubled kids. And the concept of providing health care in schools is now part of mainstream policy thinking. But if making a difference implies something on a larger scale, then school-based clinics have fallen short of the mark.

With the devolution of social programs to state and local governments in the 1980s, the federal government could no longer be counted on to expand successful demonstration programs. The changed social and political environment led the Foundation to modify its approach and to begin working directly with state and local governments and developing partnerships with community groups. Rather than testing and evaluating models, the Foundation now looks to fund programs that engage the community, are large enough to meet the need, and will continue after the Foundation's funding ends. How has it gone about developing programs based on these principles? What factors have influenced the Foundation?

- *The quality of a program's leadership.* This determines whether a program will be able to engage the community and formulate a vision. It is therefore crucial to identify local leaders and allow them the freedom to identify problems and formulate appropriate strategies. The Urban Health Initiative (1995 to 2002), for example, which is designed to improve child health outcomes in entire cities, does not fund particular programs. Rather, by encouraging community leaders to spearhead the push for reform, it supports leadership training for local organizers, who tend to be former public officials or executives of charitable organizations. The idea is that these participants will tap into their professional and personal networks to raise funds and recruit staff to effect change—and, just as important, that members of an existing local power structure will come to have a stake in making the program work and continuing it even after the Robert Wood Johnson grant ends. In fact, some recent Foundation programs have focused not on providing a specific service but on leadership training and community mobilization.

- *Collaboration among local leaders.* If local leaders cooperate in determining what needs to be done and in committing resources to support a plan, the program is more likely to succeed and last. One of the most important tasks the collaborative effort can carry out is to identify and involve influential players in the public and private sectors in order to alter systems in a way that will support long-term change and sustain new approaches. If influential constituencies are involved from the beginning, the program is more likely to attract funding from local agencies, and thus to last beyond the term of the Foundation's grant. This principle has informed the approach taken by the Urban Health Initiative. The Foundation required that applicants submit a "single letter of interest" reflecting the contributions of many community organizations, so that collaboration between groups that might not have previously worked together could be established from the start. By involving community leaders at the outset, the Urban Health Initiative is expected to build a constituency that has a stake in sustaining the program.

- *Community participation.* Being too prescriptive with grantees may help reach a program's goals in the short term but sabotage it in the long term. In the Foundation's early days, it tended to develop relatively rigid guidelines so that, much like a clinical trial of a new drug, approaches to problems could be evaluated and compared: for the project on the regionalization of perinatal care, it developed a standard risk assessment to determine which mothers-to-be required transport to a perinatal center; for the Rural Infant Care Program, The Robert Wood Johnson Foundation

defined precisely the population to be served; with the Infant
Health and Development Program, the day care curriculum was
defined down to the toys available. With David Olds's program to
have nurses visit pregnant women at home, too, the Foundation
specified the frequency of visits and the services the nurses would
offer the mothers. One risk of conducting such scientific studies,
however, is that programs could be viewed as "belonging" to the
Foundation, and not to the community. Without a feeling of ownership, a political entity appears less likely to allocate scarce
resources to a new program; without the feeling that a community
is guiding a program, there is no public pressure to continue it
once the Foundation ends its support.

This realization has shaped the more recent Foundation-supported programs in children's health. The Urban Health Initiative
offers the best example of this. The application process for the
Urban Health Initiative, for instance, asked grantees, "What factors most influence the health and safety of the children in your
area?" The answers, and the choices for how to use the grants,
have sometimes been surprising: the most frequent responses cite
violence, poor education, and the lack of meaningful (and safe)
after-school and weekend activities for children. The result has
been an impressive diversity of programs. In Philadelphia, the
program's leaders concluded that having no place but the streets
or unsupervised homes to return to after school posed one of the
greatest threats to their children; they chose to establish after-
school centers with sports, art, and mentoring programs. Urban
Health Initiative leaders in Baltimore are working with the police
chief and the district attorney to establish an antigang program
modeled on a successful program in Boston. In Richmond, the
program's leaders are helping schools figure out ways to get every
child reading by third grade. Detroit's leaders used the Urban
Health Initiative to establish a mentoring program; by linking
volunteers and children who are at risk for substance abuse and
dropping out, these community leaders believed that they could
do more for the health of Detroit's children than, say, a more traditional health program such as asthma screening. In Oakland,
the leaders are simply trying to get children to and from school
safely; they have established a neighborhood watch plan whose
linchpin is placing police officers in drug-ridden public housing
projects.

• *Partnerships with public or other agencies.* The National Council on Aging's Family Friends Program paired older volunteers with chronically ill children and their families, and continued years after the Foundation's 6 years of support ended, in 1991. In addition to being sustained at its original sites in eight cities, Family Friends expanded to new cities. The Rural Infant Care Program funded ten medical schools for a collaboration with local and state health agencies to reduce infant mortality in isolated rural areas. Although university faculty members made themselves less available to the projects after the Foundation's support ended, that did not necessarily spell the end of the effort; the state of Oklahoma and some counties in other states continued to fund the program, and local health departments took over six sites. In Yakima, Washington, the formation of a regional perinatal care steering committee made up of local leaders and of officials from the state health department allowed the Rural Infant Care Program to stay alive. In all cases, the program endured by cultivating a base of political and bureaucratic support. Similarly, Healthy Children (1983 to 1990), a program to develop new children's services, especially school-based health services, set up some two dozen clinics. The American Academy of Pediatrics took over the program, recruiting "facilitators" from 56 of the Academy's 59 chapters. This commitment was the key to sustainability.

• *Paying attention to political turf and targeting the right level of government.* The Child Health Initiative—the pilot program to decategorize funds—offers a clear example of this. The Foundation awarded grants to six local governments (Marion County, Oregon; Minneapolis; Monroe County, New York; San Francisco; Scott County, Iowa; Seattle/King County), one state agency (in Miller County, Arkansas), and two nonprofit community groups (in Cumberland County, Maine, and in Flint, Michigan). Each was to pool existing funds for children's health programs and lift restrictions on the use of categorical funds so that health services for (usually) impoverished and often chronically ill children would be delivered more efficiently. A typical patient might be a 15-year-old diabetic who also abuses alcohol and is sexually active. She needs inpatient care to control her diabetes, treatment for alcoholism, and family planning services.

Her family is ineligible for Medicaid but has no health insurance. Eligibility criteria for available programs (Maternal and Child Health block grant programs, lead screening, mental health services, WIC) differ, as do enrollment procedures and reimbursement policies. In short, there is a bureaucratic morass that few families can wade through.

According to an evaluation by a team led by Paul Newacheck of the Institute for Health Policy Studies of the University of California at San Francisco, not a single Child Health Initiative site managed to create a pool of flexible funds out of money from categorical programs; only Monroe County made any progress toward that goal by trying to decategorize the multiple funding streams from state and federal programs. What went wrong? On the tactical level, Newacheck says, the Foundation failed to provide clear guidance to the sites. It prepared no formal documents to describe the purpose or the expectations of the projects. A change in leadership at the program's national office left grantees without daily guidance for several months, Newacheck found, and "created an information vacuum." But there were larger, strategic problems, too.

Decategorization requires support from those with the authority to grant exemptions or waivers from categorical programs such as those for maternal and child health care; these people are generally in state or federal offices, but the project was largely confined to the local level, which Newacheck says was "probably a mistake." Asking a locality to lead the effort to decategorize funds is like giving Sisyphus shoes with better traction: the task is still nearly impossible because of the typically weak relationships between local staff and higher-level policy makers who run the programs and control the money. "Placing responsibility at the local level to achieve decategorization without connections to the state and federal policy level placed the sites at a distinct disadvantage," the evaluation team concluded.[15] "High level political commitments to the effort are needed between all levels of government." Otherwise, turf and control issues trump recognition of what might be best for the recipients of services.

Even at the local level, turf battles flared. Decategorization, by definition, wrests control of funds from particular agencies and individuals. The department in charge of, say, substance abuse

treatment wasn't thrilled about siphoning off part of its budget
into a general pool of funds to be administered by someone else.
Agencies wanted assurance that their own clients would receive
special consideration when funds were decategorized. Monroe
County was the only site to achieve even partial success, because
the funds it targeted for decategorization were administered
through its own health department—that is, the grantee itself.
The project director was the director of the health department.
The state health department signed on to the cause, and the
county retained consultants who facilitated negotiations with
the federal government to waive categorical restrictions on the
use of funds.

The Covering Kids program, too, acknowledges the importance of involving stakeholders and building political coalitions.
To apply for funding, each state had to form a coalition and des-
ignate a single agency to lead it; that lead agency could be anything from the state health agency or a state medical association
to a child advocacy group, a religious association, or a philanthropy. But involving the agencies that have the power to effect
change or thwart it was critical. "The old idea was that states
have been slow to help the poor, so you need strong outside
advocates to get anything done," says Michael Rothman, a senior
program officer at the Foundation, who had worked previously
in the Colorado governor's office. "But we've learned that you
have to engage the decision makers." With as many players as
possible given a stake in the program's success, bureaucratic hurdles would be lowered and turf battles minimized.

• *Developing larger programs.* The Foundation is urging more and
more of its grantees to think of meeting children's needs in an
entire city or area. "We're actually having some success in changing the mindset that going from 100 kids to 200 counts as a tri-
umph," Foundation vice president Paul Jellinek says. Program
officers of the Urban Health Initiative have been relentless in
hammering home the idea that it is time to help *all* the kids in a
city—creating some bad feelings in agencies that aren't used to
thinking this way. But, slowly, grantees are recognizing that their
approaches are too narrow. "We are trying to leverage change,"
Jellinek says. "Of course, the amount of the grant isn't nearly
enough"—enough, that is to improve the health or health care

of a city's entire population of kids. "But we are getting people to see that setting up after-school programs in three or four schools is a non-starter if it's going to reach no more than 5 percent of your kids. So instead of working to convince a few principals to institute the program, we're showing grantees that they need to change the policy at the level of the school system. They need to work to keep schools open after hours, to train volunteers, to involve the parks and recreation department and the faith community." The program thus becomes a challenge of a different magnitude, and one that service agencies are generally unaccustomed to. But that's why the Urban Health Initiative supported only coalitions that showed signs of being able to push for change at this level.

Beyond modifying its programs to adapt to the changed social and political environment, the Foundation has recognized the importance of giving program managers the flexibility to deal with unforeseen economic changes and new market forces. Without this flexibility, even successful programs vetted by sound scientific assessments can founder. Consider one of the Foundation's earliest children's health efforts, the Regionalized Perinatal Care Program. The goal was to make the then-emerging technologies of caring for high-risk fetuses and newborns, especially premature babies, available to women regardless of where they lived. The program was therefore funded from 1975 to 1983 to organize hospital collaborations so that expensive perinatal technologies could be shared. Eight sites received a total of $17.6 million to test regionalization: three areas in Los Angeles, the Upper West Side of Manhattan, Arizona, Cuyahoga County in Ohio, Dallas County in Texas, and 15 counties around Syracuse, New York. The results in both the study regions and the comparison regions were positive but not appreciably different from one another: neonatal mortality in the study regions fell 19 percent from 1974 or 1975 to 1978 or 1979, and by 25 percent in the comparison areas. One feared consequence of saving preemies was that the babies would survive only to be forever handicapped. But this, by and large, did not occur in the short term. In fact, at one year of age, the percentage of low-birthweight babies with disabilities had decreased, and the program could boast of "graduates" like Adam Gensel, born four weeks early in 1978 and weighing only 4 pounds, 1 ounce. After his mother was admitted to her local hospital in Painesville, Ohio, in her 36th week of pregnancy with high blood pressure and a smaller than normal uterus, she was transferred to University Hospitals of Cleveland, part of the Cleveland Regional Perinatal Network. Adam spent his first 13 days in the neonatal intensive care unit. He went home in good condition, and had a normal, healthy childhood.[16]

The Regionalized Perinatal Care Program met its stated goal of furthering hospital collaborations and reducing infant mortality, but fell short of the Foundation's expectation that it would make a lasting difference. After Foundation support ended, few of the regional compacts endured. Perhaps this should not have come as a surprise: after all, regionalization meant that a woman's primary hospital not only would lose a paying patient but also would see a decline in its caseload. (Caseload helps determine reimbursement eligibility under state and federal regulations.) But regionalization faced two other hurdles. First, with an increasing number of perinatologists, the idea of placing neonatal intensive care units only into sophisticated, tertiary care hospitals fell by the wayside; other hospitals, too, began establishing neonatal intensive care units and competing for patients with the tertiary care hospitals. Second, it ran smack into the onslaught of managed care, with its networks of physicians and hospitals determining more than any other factors where a woman would deliver her baby. Competition reduced the willingness of physicians and hospitals to cooperate in establishing an integrated perinatal health care system. The 1992 evaluation of the Foundation's maternal and child health grants concluded, "The competitive environment of today has undermined many aspects of the perinatal regionalization."[17] To have a meaningful and lasting effect on children's health, the Foundation must understand—and even anticipate—changes in health care policy and practice, such as the push to enroll Medicaid patients in managed care.

Over the years, the Foundation has learned the value of supporting programs and people that push health and health care beyond the boundaries of the clinic. The Foundation recognized from its inception that health neither begins nor ends at the provider's office, but instead exists against a backdrop of socioeconomic status and the larger culture. Children's health, in other words, means more than medical care. "The factors contributing to so many of the disorders we label 'health problems' are part of the social and economic fabric of families and communities," an evaluation team led by Dr. Robert J. Haggerty concluded in 1992, citing an estimate that only 25 percent of changes in child health occur as a result of medical services.[18]

Although this was hardly mainstream thinking, respected medical professionals suggested ways of going well beyond the walls of the clinic. In 1988 Dr. Margaret Heagarty, chief of pediatrics at Harlem Hospital, sought support for a program she had launched that aimed at reducing the number of emergency room admissions. Dr. Heagarty had an unusual way of achieving that: she wanted to get neighborhood kids into Little League, to clean glass out of playgrounds, to put bars on apartment windows—in other words, to take actions that do not usually qualify as "health care." The Foundation supported her initial effort, and the program grew into the Injury-Free Coalition for Kids (1988 to 1992 and 1994 to 1997). Led by Dr. Barbara Barlow, director of pediatric surgical services at Harlem Hospital, this program established a number of after-school programs, among them art, gardening, bicycle repair, and fencing. Barlow also created a home-safety checklist, warning parents about household poisons, kitchen burns, and windows that lack safety bars. In the first year of the program, Harlem Hospital's emergency room admissions of children fell 55 percent. In the years from 1988 to 1992, admission to Harlem Hospital's emergency room because of children's injuries decreased by 41 percent, compared with baseline data gathered for the period 1983 to 1988.

The Foundation funded similar projects in five other cities, each of which also used a greatly expanded definition of health. The Chicago program, at the Cabrini Green and Washington Park housing projects, also distributed a home-safety checklist; in addition, it recruited volunteers to teach kids ballet, reading, computers, science, and other topics, with the goal of preventing street violence and teenage pregnancy. Girls who stayed in the program were three times as likely to graduate from high school, and to avoid jail and pregnancy, as girls who dropped out.

The Foundation has also learned that there is no single right approach to improving children's health and that it must tailor its approaches—in some instances, funding categorical programs, in other instances more comprehensive programs—depending on the circumstances. "Categorical" means interventions for a single need; "comprehensive" describes a range of services given over the years to the same high-risk child. Because the risks that children face do not exist in isolation, "it is illogical, inefficient, and ineffective to devise programs that address each problem separately," concludes a report on 20 years of Robert Wood Johnson Foundation grant making.[19] Indeed, many of the more recent programs—particularly those intended to reach children living within a certain geographic area—are designed to offer a wide range of services. The Nurse Home Visiting Program of David Olds is one of the longest-established examples of the comprehensive approach. More recent examples are the Urban Health Initiative and the Injury Free Coalition for Kids. All of these offer a wide range of services—some of them clinical but many of them nonmedical. Still, this does not represent the totality of the Foundation's approach. It recently funded a program to test different ways to reduce asthma, and its All Kids Count program focused exclusively on immunization—both of them categorical programs focused on a single problem.

⸻ Conclusion

Programs to promote children's health have increased steadily during the lifetime of the Foundation: in 1972, they accounted for 11 percent of total grants, while in 1997 they accounted for 35 percent. But the increase in numbers is only part of the story. The other part is how the programs have evolved. From the well-controlled demonstrations that characterized the Foundation's early years, the Foundation has moved to larger, more wide-ranging approaches that attempt to remove financial barriers to obtaining care, work to provide multiple services to defined population of kids, and, through a new center that is currently in the exploration stage, to make the latest knowledge about children's health available to families and policy makers. The kinds of programs that now receive support—enrolling children in Medicaid with Covering Kids, building coalitions of businessmen and politicians with the Urban Health Initiative, supporting after-school programs with the Injury Free Coalition for Kids—would hardly be recognizable to a children's health program officer of a quarter century ago. They reflect both the way in which The Robert Wood Johnson Foundation has adapted to the changing social environment and the tenacity needed to achieve an important goal—improving the health and well-being of children.

Notes

1. The program is examined by M. Holloway in this *Anthology*.
2. M. C. McCormick et al. "The Health and Developmental Status of Very Low-Birth-Weight Children at School Age." *The Journal of the American Medical Association*, 1992, *267*(16), 2204–2208.

3. These were the Bureau of Community Health Services, Commonwealth Fund, Ford Foundation, National Center for Nursing Research, National Institutes of Health, and the W.T. Grant Foundation.

4. D. Olds et al. "Long Term Effects of Home Visitation on Maternal Life Course and Child Abuse and Neglect: 15-year Follow-up of a Randomized Trial." *The Journal of the American Medical Association*, 1997, *278*(8), 637–643, D. Olds et al. "Long Term Effects of Nurse Home Visitation on Children's Criminal and Antisocial Behavior: 15-year Follow-up of a Randomized Controlled Trial." *The Journal of the American Medical Association*, 1998, *280*(14), 1238–1244.

5. L. A. Karoly et al. *Investing in Our Children: What We Know and Don't Know About the Costs and Benefits of Early Childhood Interventions.* Santa Monica, Calif.: The RAND Corporation, 1998.

6. The Foundation's work in school-based health is examined in Paul Brodeur, "School-Based Health Clinics." In S. L. Isaacs and J. R. Knickman, (eds.), *To Improve Health and Health Care 2000: The Robert Wood Johnson Foundation Anthology.* San Francisco: Jossey-Bass, 1999.

7. J. G. Lear, N. Eichner, and J. Koppelman. "The Growth of School-Based Health Centers and the Role of State Policies: Results of a National Survey." *Archives of Pediatrics and Adolescent Medicine*, 1999, *153*(11), 1177–1180; and H. Lee. "Overview of Public Elementary and Secondary Schools and Districts: School Year 1997–1998." *Education Statistics Quarterly*, 1999, *1*(3).

8. This is examined in M. Holloway, "Expanding Health Insurance for Children," in S. L. Isaacs and J. R. Knickman (eds.), *To Improve Health and Health Care 2000: The Robert Wood Johnson Foundation Anthology.* San Francisco: Jossey-Bass, 1999.

9. S. Basalla. *Twenty-Five Years of Children's Health Grantmaking 1972–1997.* The Robert Wood Johnson Foundation Internal Report, June, 1998, p. 39.

10. All Kids Count is examined in G. DeFriese et al. "Developing Child Immunization Registries: The All Kids Count Program." In S. L. Isaacs and J. R. Knickman, (eds.), *To Improve Health and Health Care 1997: The Robert Wood Johnson Foundation Anthology.* San Francisco: Jossey-Bass, 1997.

11. The program is examined in L. Saxe and T. P. Cross, "The Mental Health Services Program for Youth." In S. L. Isaacs and J. R. Knickman, (eds.), *To Improve Health and Health Care 1998–1999: The Robert Wood Johnson Foundation Anthology.* San Francisco: Jossey-Bass, 1998.

12. Ibid, p. 175.

13. P. Newacheck, N. Halfon, C. D. Brindis, and D. Hughes. "Evaluating Community Efforts to Decategorize and Integrate Financing of Children's Health Services." *Milbank Quarterly*, 1998, *76*(2), 157–173.

14. R. Haggerty and B. Guyer. *Evaluation of Grants Made 1972–1992 in Maternal and Child Health*, The Robert Wood Johnson Foundation Internal Report, November, 1992, p. 13.

15. P. Newacheck, D. Hughes, C. Brindis, and N. Halfon. "Decategorizing Health Services: Interim Findings From The Robert Wood Johnson Foundation's Child Health Initiative." *Health Affairs*, 1995, *14*(3), 232–242.

16. The Robert Wood Johnson Foundation, *The Perinatal Program: What Has Been Learned*, Special Report Number 3, 1985, p. 11.

17. Haggerty and Guyer 1992, op. cit., p. 25.

18. Ibid, page 51.

19. T. Cooper, et al. *Twenty Years of the Foundation Grantmaking: Five Expert Assessments*, The Robert Wood Johnson Foundation Internal Report, January, 1993, p. 54.

CHAPTER FOUR

⟿ The Changing Approach to Managed Care

Janet Firshein and Lewis G. Sandy

Editors' Introduction

The rise of managed care in the early 1970s coincided with the establishment of The Robert Wood Johnson Foundation as a national philanthropy. It is not surprising, therefore, that the Foundation has been involved, almost since its beginning, in trying to develop and shape this mechanism for financing and delivering health care services. This chapter traces the ways The Robert Wood Johnson Foundation has approached managed care over the past 29 years and illustrates how the Foundation's strategies have changed as the concept of managed care itself has evolved.

The Foundation was an early supporter of the idea that later became known as managed care. In the 1970s, it promoted the idea of prepaid group health plans by funding a number of pioneers who were experimenting with alternative systems for financing and delivering health services—the early forms of health maintenance organizations. Later, as new forms of managed care became dominant and as concerns surfaced about whether large for-profit managed care organizations were cutting costs by providing less than high-quality services and by avoiding people with chronic illness, the Foundation adjusted its strategies to address these issues. In keeping with its priorities, in the 1990s, the Foundation began to fund programs that would demonstrate how HMOs could prevent and treat alcohol, drug, and tobacco abuse among their members.

The chapter's co-authors are Janet Firshein and Lewis Sandy. Ms. Firshein, the former editor of *Medicine and Health*, is a free-lance writer who has been covering health care policy issues for 13 years. Dr. Sandy, an internist who also has an MBA, is the executive vice president of The Robert Wood Johnson Foundation. Previously, he was a physician-manager at the Harvard Community Health Plan.

—◊◊◊—

With the influence that managed care has on health care delivery today, it's hard to remember the world before it came along. Over the past three decades, managed care has gained what appears to be an enduring foothold in the American health care system. By the end of 1999, nearly 170 million people were enrolled in some form of managed care; this includes 7.1 million Medicare beneficiaries and 13.3 million poor Americans covered by Medicaid.[1] Three decades earlier, slightly more than 3 million insured Americans were enrolled in managed care plans, nearly all of them in health maintenance organizations, or HMOs.[2]

The evolution of managed care has had profound effects on health care delivery and financing in the United States. Once an obscure outgrowth of a predominately fee-for-service, retrospective payment system, managed care has, over the years, catalyzed the growth of large integrated delivery systems and squeezed excess dollars out of the health care spending pie. In the process, it has transformed traditional health care relationships and turned health care reimbursement and delivery on its head. Managed care has been the force behind efforts to improve health outcomes, mostly by encouraging wider use of preventive and primary care. Simultaneously, however, it has been vilified for restricting patients' access to their doctors and diminishing quality—all in the quest to cut health care costs.

About three-quarters of insured Americans now belong to some form of managed care arrangement, which range from more restrictive HMOs to looser preferred provider organization networks and other HMO hybrids. Nevertheless, surveys reveal that the managed care sector is second only to the tobacco industry in public distrust.

As a philanthropy, The Robert Wood Johnson Foundation has never staked out a position on the merits of managed care. But it has had a hand in shaping its development and direction over the last quarter of the twentieth century. Since the Foundation's inception, in 1972, it has spent more than $207 million on managed care–related activities. The Foundation's investment in managed care can best be viewed in evolutionary terms. Managed care originated as a single species: the nonprofit, prepaid group practice. Stimulated in part by cost inflation, the original species grew and matured. But hardier breeds—for-profit health plans—tended to be more financially robust and aggressive competitors, with access to much needed capital. These fitter species grew to dominate the health care landscape as well as to shape it.

⎯ The Origin of the Species

Modern managed care began with the industrialist Henry J. Kaiser and Dr. Sidney Garfield's innovation for meeting the needs of the builders of the Grand Coulee Dam in 1937 and of World War II shipyard and steel workers—the prepaid group practice. The California-based Kaiser Permanente was organized in 1945 to promote a new kind of health care delivery that was built around medical groups and prepaid, capitated financing. By organizing medical care within physician groups, these pioneers felt that they could improve the continuity and the quality of care, encourage providers to constrain expenses when possible, and avoid overutilizing services.

In spite of the opposition of organized medicine, which viewed these arrangements as a step toward socialized medicine, Kaiser and other prepaid group practices, such as the Group Health Cooperative of Puget Sound, continued to grow. Their integrated delivery systems and unique financing allowed them to provide less expensive medical care than fee-for-service insurance. This cost advantage, modest in absolute terms when health insurance represented a small fraction of employee benefit costs, proved crucial for HMO growth and policy influence.

By the late 1960s, rising health care expenditures encouraged employers to make wider use of HMOs. Paul Ellwood, Jr., then an aide to President Richard Nixon, coined the term "health maintenance organization" in 1970. Ellwood, a physician, believed that restructuring the financing of health care into a capitated system that would reward providers for maintaining patients' health would improve outcomes and lower health costs. Thus, the Nixon Administration moved to develop a health policy framework around HMOs, culminating in the HMO Act of 1973. Nixon and his aides envisioned a rapid expansion of HMOs as a way to curb health inflation and redirect medical care toward preventing rather than just treating illness. The Act lifted barriers to HMO development, helping the expansion along by requiring businesses with more than 25 workers to offer an HMO option, if available, as an alternative to traditional coverage. The Act also provided grants and loans to start new HMOs.

In 1971, fewer than 4 million Americans were enrolled in nearly 40 prepaid health plans, most of which were operating in California.[3] The Nixon Administration expected to create nearly 1,700 HMOs. Nixon's staff optimistically forecast that by 1980 some 90 percent of the American population would have access to an HMO.[4]

—— First Steps: Planting New Seeds for Development

It was in this environment that The Robert Wood Johnson Foundation began operating as a national philanthropy. Its leaders believed that national health insurance was on the horizon, and that organized group practices that emphasized cost-effective primary care would help meet the nation's need to assure access, control costs, and improve quality. The Foundation, then headed by the late David Rogers, decided it should help direct the future of prepaid group practice by cultivating and nourishing academically based prepaid group practices.

Given the major federal impetus to promote HMO development, the decision was a logical step. The medical schools, after all, train the next generation of providers. It was thought crucial for schools to develop the ability to prepare young physicians for this new delivery mode. Moreover, since prepaid group practices emphasized primary care, academically affiliated HMOs could help increase the supply of primary care providers by serving as sites for ambulatory training.

Rogers was no stranger to prepaid health care. Before coming to the Foundation, he was dean of The Johns Hopkins University School of Medicine and the founder of the Hopkins Plan, a prepaid group practice model. Robert Blendon, a professor at the Harvard University School of Public Health who worked with Rogers at Johns Hopkins and then at the Foundation, says the University's plan and others like it had developed effective ways of practicing medicine that were worthy of exploration and encouragement. Having physicians work within a budget in which they could decide patient care priorities "was seen as a promising alternative," he says. This was a new organizational form, a place to train the next generation of health care professionals on how to practice in this environment.

One of the earliest initiatives undertaken by The Robert Wood Johnson Foundation was to help the Boston-based Harvard Community Health Plan. Harvard had had a site downtown, but it had reached enrollment capacity. In the early 1970s, the Foundation gave

Harvard Community Health Plan about $1 million to fund the start-up of a second health center in Cambridge, Massachusetts. The creation of a center in Cambridge was an attempt by the Harvard Community Health Plan to expand its reach in the metropolitan area. Harvard was a safe investment for a lot of reasons. It had strong ties to the Harvard Medical School. Dean Robert Ebert advocated a stronger role for Harvard in the education of primary care physicians, and looked to the health plan to provide leadership in this area.

The Foundation also provided support to other less developed plans, including Georgetown University's Community Health plan and the Yale New Haven Community Health Center, and gave $350,000 in seed money to the Martinez Health Center in Martinez, California, to develop an HMO.

This initial grant making undoubtedly helped these fledgling health plans, but HMO development turned out to be a daunting task. The Martinez Center, which cared for an underserved population, had trouble attracting enrollees. After one year of operation, only about 1,000 people had enrolled, and the Foundation did not provide additional support. Yale New Haven also had its problems, with enrollment falling below projections and deficits growing higher than anticipated. The Foundation terminated its support for this project as well. The Foundation supported the Georgetown plan much longer, spending a total of $631,000 over eight years to assist with start-up costs and other operating expenses. But in 1980, that grant ended as well.

By the end of the 1970s, HMOs did not dominate the health care system. Instead, they remained in a contained niche. It became clear that starting up and operating HMOs was an extraordinarily complex and expensive endeavor. In addition, most physicians preferred solo or small group practice. And the Nixonian vision for HMO expansion had not panned out.

By late 1979, there were fewer than 250 HMOs on the market—far fewer than Nixon had anticipated.[5] Only about 4 percent of the population, or 8 million people, were enrolled in these plans.[6] By the early 1980s, other pressing issues were bubbling to the surface. Health care inflation was engulfing the nation, particularly in the Medicare and Medicaid programs. President Ronald Reagan began block-granting public health programs, and health policy leaders—acknowledging the failure of federal health planning laws to contain capacity and control health costs—focused on new cost-containment approaches, such as Diagnosis-Related Group, or DRG, payments for hospital care.

National health insurance seemed as elusive as ever, and the HMO movement, while growing, was clearly not the magic bullet that many had assumed it would be.

During the early and mid-1980s, the Foundation intensified its focus on increasing people's access to medical services and reducing health care costs. It supported research and demonstration projects to find out what was driving health care inflation and to test the effectiveness of cost-containment experiments directed at hospitals, physicians, and other providers.

⟶ A New Species—The For-Profit HMO

By the early 1980s, the HMO movement seemed to have lost momentum. But a new species arose—some might say by mutation; others, by invasion. Entrepreneurs—impressed with the cost savings generated by capitated, prepaid financing—saw an opportunity for a profitable business venture. With health care costs soaring at double-digit rates each year, they reasoned that it wouldn't take much to reduce health care utilization, offer a cheaper insurance product to employer groups, provide adequate medical care, and keep surpluses as profit. Through these ventures, the new players thought they could cut the number of excess hospital beds and providers and make the health care system more efficient. These new entrants, rather than create their own delivery systems, began building networks of contractual relations with hospitals and doctors.

This latest variant of HMO was a different breed from its predecessors. Predominantly for-profit, the new HMO did not emerge out of the social ethos of earlier pioneers and was not anchored in a reform of the delivery system. Like many private sector innovations, it found a need and filled it—the need for employers to control their health care expenditures.

It was during this growth phase that the health policy community began to question whether the cost savings demonstrated by managed care were the result of enrolling lower-cost, healthier people (favorable selection), reducing reimbursement to providers, improving efficiency and effectiveness, denying services, or combinations of these factors. Employers also began to ask questions. As more workers began to enroll in managed care, employers wanted to ensure that health plans were providing quality services and appropriate access. They began to develop customized, detailed contracts requiring that data on quality be reported. Each employer had different requirements. HMOs began

Table 4.1.   Glossary of Terms.

Term	Definition
Ambulatory Care	All types of health services that are provided on an outpatient basis in contrast to services provided in the home or for inpatients in health care institutions. In other words, health services provided without admitting the patient to a hospital or long-term care facility.
Block Grants	Grant funds made to local and state government units by the federal government. Although states are required to submit an annual plan explaining how such funds will be used, there is great flexibility in the distribution of grant money as long as the funds are used for acceptable purposes.
Capitation	A method of payment for health services in which an individual or institutional provider is paid a fixed, per capita amount for each person served without regard to the actual number or nature of services provided to each person. Capitation is a set money amount received or paid out, usually under a contract, and is paid in advance on the basis of membership enrollments rather than on services delivered.
Diagnosis-Related Group (DRG)	An approach to classifying a patient's disease or condition and treatment procedures in terms of the expected consumption of hospital resources. Medicare began using Diagnosis-Related Groups in 1983 to reduce hospital costs by encouraging the reduction of the length of stay of patients.
Fee-For-Service	A method of charging patients for medical care services or treatment whereby a physician or other practitioner bills the insurance company or the patient for each patient encounter, treatment, or service rendered.
Group Practice	A formal association of three or more physicians or other health professionals who share expenses, facilities, staff and diagnostic equipment, lab, information management systems, and administrative overhead.
Health Maintenance Organization (HMO)	A prepaid health plan that provides comprehensive health care services for a specified group or members at a fixed cost or through prepaid periodic payments. Members are required to seek services from the health plan's set of physicians and other health practitioners, except in certain specified situations.

ꞔ𝄞ꞔ

Table 4.1.　Glossary of Terms, *continued.*

Term	Definition
Integrated Delivery System	A single organization or a group of affiliated organizations, which consists of physicians, dispersed clinic settings, hospitals, a referral network, and full continuum of after-care offerings, that provides the full range of health care services to a population of enrollees within a market area or fairly large regional area.
Preferred Provider Organization (PPO)	Specialized health care delivery organizations formed by hospitals, physicians, medical groups, or health plans that negotiate fee schedules with insurance companies, thus becoming preferred. The patient has a financial incentive—stemming from lower copayments and deductibles—to use the preferred provider.
Prepaid Group Practice	A formal association of three or more physicians or other health professionals that provides a defined set of services to persons over a specified time period in return for a fixed periodic prepayment made in advance of the use of service.
Risk Adjustment	The process of trying to compensate companies that have an unusually high number of high-cost enrollees by adjusting reimbursement for enrollee characteristics such as severity of illness.

Sources: Thomas C. Timmreck, *Health Services Cyclopedic Dictionary: A Compendium of Health-Care and Public Health Terminology,* Third Edition (Sudbury, Mass.: Jones and Bartlett Publishers, 1997) and Richard Rognehaugh, *The Managed Health Care Dictionary,* Second Edition (Gaithersburg, Md.: Aspen Publishers, 1998).

---

to stagger under the administrative burden of trying to comply with all of them. In addition, both the policy community and the public began to be concerned about the quality of care that HMOs were providing.

⎯⎯ Contributing to HMO Quality

By the late 1980s, The Robert Wood Johnson Foundation focused on this new species of HMO and began to develop programs to both improve managed care quality and better understand how the dynamics of the managed care marketplace were affecting the entire health care system. For example, as insurers, HMO finances were heavily regulated, but there was no single entity responsible for assuring that the quality of medical care for enrollees met a specific standard. Unlike hospitals and physicians, there was no recognized certifying body to accredit HMOs.

It was in this context that in 1988 the Foundation provided a small grant, of $49,000, to an obscure group called the National Committee for Quality Assurance, or NCQA. NCQA was established in the late 1970s by industry trade groups to do so-called quality review, because of the fear that the federal government might create a similar review body for HMOs that received federal funds. NCQA, however, made little progress in developing an effective quality review system, and by the late 1980s it had become moribund. The grant was meant to support a national survey of HMOs and convene a series of focus groups comprised of HMO leaders, payers, and other industry experts. The objective was to redirect NCQA's focus and assess whether there was a need for an accreditation program, whether industry would be willing to support such an effort, and whether there were sufficient methodologies in existence to develop an accreditation process.

Peter Fox, now a private consultant in Washington, D.C., who was involved in those early sessions, said the gatherings "were trying to get at whether there were enough employers who cared about the quality issue to see whether accreditation was something they would consider." He added, "There was a general feeling at the time that the only reason that an HMO would request accreditation is if employers cared about it."

In 1989, a handful of the nation's largest employers decided to insist on performance data from HMOs with whom they did business. A group of leading health plans, inundated with multiple requests for variants of similar quality data, were seeking to simplify their administrative load and keep the employers happy. Eventually, this small band of employers and health plans agreed that the proper direction was to develop one standardized set of quality measures rather than having health plans meet different benchmarks for different companies.[7] These employers and HMO leaders settled on a few standard prevention indicators that HMOs would report on, such as how often they immunized children or gave mammograms to women. These standards were called the "Health Plan Employer Data and Information Set" or HEDIS, a central mechanism to determine how well plans perform certain basic health care services. NCQA seemed like a logical place to develop this approach further.

With the assurance that an HMO certification program would be both feasible and desirable, NCQA won a second, more generous grant from the Foundation to help it develop and implement an accreditation program for HMOs. In 1990, the Foundation awarded a three-year $309,000 grant to NCQA to help it refine standards for quality review, develop a training program for accreditation reviewers, and create a marketing strategy. In an unusual move at the time, the Foundation asked that its grant be matched by the HMO industry—an important requirement because it assured that the managed care sector would support the program. That support helped establish NCQA as a viable entity. "The Foundation gave us the wherewithal to become an independent organization," says Margaret O'Kane, who has been president of NCQA since its inception.

Since 1991, NCQA has been accrediting HMOs and assessing whether health plans have the controls they need to evaluate the quality of services they deliver. Today, it is the nation's leading organization measuring quality in managed care plans. Although observers differ in their views of NCQA's influence on employer purchasing practices, most would agree that it has raised standards in the managed care industry, led health plans and payers to focus on outcomes, and forced managed care operators to examine their internal quality assurance systems.

ↄⅉℙ

Table 4.2.   National Programs on Managed Care of The Robert Wood Johnson Foundation.

Name	Years	Funding Amount*
Program for Prepaid Managed Health Care	1982–1989	$17,499,969
Chronic Care Initiatives in HMOs	1992–1997	6,945,362
Health Tracking (Center for Studying Health System Change)	1994–2002	104,737,409
Medicaid Managed Care Program	1995–2004	47,600,000
Addressing Tobacco in Managed Care	1996–2003	6,760,000
Improving Chronic Illness Care	1998–2003	25,000,000

* For closed programs, the funding amount is total spending including planning, evaluation, technical assistance, and other expenses. For active programs, the funding amount is the current authorization for implementation.

⎯⎯ Managed Care's Grip on Health Care

By the early 1990s, with health care costs still soaring and the ranks of the uninsured swelling, the managed care industry was enjoying rapid growth. Meanwhile, a growing body of health services research had documented that for the most part the quality of care in HMOs was no worse than in fee-for-service, and was better in delivering some preventive services.[8] And the cost advantage of managed care continued.

In this context, the 1992 presidential election elevated the promise of managed care. Bill Clinton promised to control health costs and assure universal access to health care by building on the theory of "managed competition," in which consumers would get their health insurance through regional purchasing cooperatives that would contract with a variety of health plans including HMOs, PPOs, and conventional insurance policies. These plans would be required to offer a minimum standard set of benefits to every enrollee, who could choose among products every year. Managed competition was a policy construct developed by a hardy band of managed care devotees who called themselves the Jackson Hole Group, because they met regularly in Paul Ellwood's living room in that picturesque Wyoming town.

The demise of the Clinton health reform initiative in 1994 created a new opportunity for managed care plans. With market forces pretty much controlling health care, employers embraced managed care as the vehicle to manage employees' health and health costs. In addition, managed care was seen as an attractive option for many Medicare beneficiaries because it offered benefits that traditional Medicare left uncovered, such as prescription drugs or hearing aids, and required nominal or no out-of-pocket contributions. The government's strategy of financing Medicare HMOs made these plans particularly profitable in high cost areas such as Florida.

State Medicaid programs, also concerned with cost, began to support voluntary, then mandatory, managed care programs for beneficiaries. Finally, hospitals and physician groups were pushed by the national health care reform debate into developing integrated delivery systems and trying to build market share. These goals were achieved by contracting with as many managed care plans as possible.

~~ The Foundation's Role— Understanding, Shaping, and Tracking

As the Foundation considered its role in improving health and health care in the early 1990s, it was obvious that managed care would have increasingly powerful effects on both health care and health policy. The for-profit HMO sector alone was taking off. In 1981, roughly 18 percent of all HMOs were for-profit. By 1995, the number had risen to 70 percent.[9]

Foundation staff speculated that managed care would finally tackle the issue of an oversupply of hospital beds, equipment, and specialists in certain areas. The tools of managed care seemed to be able to moderate health care cost increases; however, the collateral damage to vulnerable providers and patients was uncertain. Managed care's emphasis on primary care and population health supported important public health principles. But in the mid-1990s the actual performance of HMOs in delivering preventive services and coordinated care began to be questioned.[10]

Throughout the 1990s, the Foundation's approach to managed care was aimed at seeking to understand how various system changes affected people; at seizing opportunities to shape critical aspects of managed care delivery; and at tracking how the health care system was evolving in a dynamic market environment.

~~ Addressing Chronically Ill Enrollees

One of the biggest unknowns about managed care has been its effect on the ability of people with chronic medical conditions to get adequate care. With a growing number of Americans joining HMOs, it became clear that there was a dearth of systematic research on how they provide care for chronically ill patients. The Foundation felt that health plans were not directing enough of their focus to people with chronic conditions, yet with their emphasis on wellness and prevention, they had the incentive to help chronically ill people better manage their conditions.

In 1989, the Foundation contracted with the consulting firm of Lewin/ICF to compile data on HMO initiatives for chronically ill seniors. The project, done in collaboration with the University of Colorado and the Group Health Association of America (now the American Association of Health Plans), showed that the bulk of large

HMOs had not developed comprehensive care programs that targeted the special needs of the chronically ill. A workshop was convened to set a research and demonstration agenda linked to caring for elderly people in a prepaid setting. This workshop was significant because for the first time it brought together leading researchers in the fields of geriatrics and health services with leaders of the HMO industry.

By 1991, with more than 36 million Americans in HMOs and a growing number of Medicaid and Medicare enrollees being channeled into these plans,[11] the Foundation decided that HMOs were likely to be enrolling increasing numbers of chronically ill patients. Moreover, HMOs could be useful settings for exploring new ways of organizing and delivering care to individuals with chronic health care needs. Because of capitation, HMOs could, in theory, reallocate resources from expensive marginally usefully tests and procedures toward low-technology services that could improve functioning and quality of life for chronically ill patients. As a result, HMOs could become the catalyst for changing practice in this area of medicine.

So in 1992, with a $5.6 million authorization, the Foundation began the Chronic Care Initiatives in HMOs, a four-year program designed to provide HMO managers, medical directors, providers, and payers with research and practice data to guide them in paying for and delivering chronic care services.[12] Overall, the project was meant to identify, nurture, and evaluate methods by which HMOs recognized high-risk chronically ill people for special interventions; to understand the impact of case management in the HMO setting (an area where there was virtually no research); and to figure out better ways to deliver primary care services in both nursing homes and ambulatory care settings.

The program supported some significant activities, including helping the NCQA develop chronic care benchmarks to incorporate into their HEDIS measures. Under the program, in 1994, The Robert Wood Johnson Foundation provided an $86,099 grant to NCQA to help it develop performance measures designed to assess how well HMOs care for enrollees with chronic illnesses. In 1996, it provided a $636,893 grant to the same accrediting group to develop, test, and evaluate health plan performance measures for diabetes, major depression, childhood asthma, and coronary artery disease. Both of these grants enabled NCQA to develop performance measures in these areas. All of those chronic conditions are part of HEDIS 2000.

The project also supported a $609,131 project at Group Health Cooperative of Puget Sound, which developed and evaluated a new approach to providing managed primary care to patients with chronic conditions within specialized chronic care clinics.

Another initiative was to create the HMO Work Group on Care, comprised of health plan leaders. The Work Group created a special screening tool to assist managed care systems identify upon enrollment senior members at high risk of frequent hospitalization. The Blue Cross and Blue Shield Association has recommended its use by managed care plans that enroll Medicare beneficiaries, and more than 50 health plans have begun using this instrument.

Based on the experience of the Chronic Care Initiatives in HMOs program, it became clear that improvement in care for the chronically ill requires fundamental changes in delivery systems. Relations between primary care and specialists need to be rethought; information systems that can track and distribute information over time and at multiple sites need to be in place, and teams of providers need to attend to the multiple medical and social needs of patients and their families.

To move the field forward, the Foundation authorized $25 million in 1998 for a five-year national program based at the Center for Health Studies at the Group Health Cooperative of Puget Sound, building on the work of a Chronic Care Initiatives grantee, Edward H. Wagner, a leader in the field of chronic care. The Program for Improving Chronic Illness Care is under the direction of Wagner, who also heads the Mac-Coll Institute for Healthcare Innovation. The goal of the program is to identify and test innovative ways to help health care systems treat chronically ill patients. The program will assist up to 120 health care systems design, implement, and evaluate state-of-the-art disease management projects, focusing on such conditions as diabetes, depression, and congestive heart failure. Since this project is still in the early phases, it's premature to draw conclusions about its overall impact at this point.

⎯⎯ Making Managed Care Work for Medicaid Recipients

In the early 1990s, managed care—with its promise of significant cost savings—was increasingly viewed as an attractive option by state leaders eager to slow the growth of Medicaid expenditures and cover more of their uninsured residents.

Mandatory use of managed care by Medicaid recipients exploded in the early 1990s. By 1995, 11.6 million Medicaid beneficiaries—a third of the program population—were enrolled in a managed care plan.[13] Twelve years earlier, only about 750,000 beneficiaries out of a pool of 22 million were enrolled in managed care.[14] The managed care phenomenon represented a sea change in the way the United States delivered care to the poor, the disabled, and the chronically ill who were covered by Medicaid. Most managed care organizations cared for employed populations, and earlier forays into Medicaid managed care—such as in California in the 1970s—were disasters. While the Foundation did not view its role as promoting or endorsing managed care, it did want to play a major role in helping to ensure that this delivery mode bolstered access to and quality of care for Medicaid beneficiaries, and did not simply save the Medicaid program money.

The Foundation's concerns were heightened by the action of Tennessee, which rushed nearly overnight into establishing its controversial TennCare program, described at the time as one of the most ambitious health care initiatives in the nation. Stephen Somers, who was a Foundation officer at the time and had a background in care for needy populations, says TennCare "was a harbinger that Medicaid managed care was going to sweep across the country and transform care for low-income people." TennCare began with minimal planning, and almost immediately faced problems with beneficiary enrollment and provider participation. Robert Wood Johnson Foundation staff members were concerned about the technical ability of states to design, implement, and monitor large-scale managed care programs, particularly those enrolling large numbers of Medicaid beneficiaries. The TennCare model—while extreme—was emblematic of that problem.

So in 1995, the Foundation established the Medicaid Managed Care Program, a national initiative under the umbrella of the Princeton-based Center for Health Care Strategies. Led by Somers, who left the Foundation to run it, the program would provide technical assistance and grants to states and managed care plans to help them identify, design, and test new models for organizing, delivering, and paying for managed care. The program was structured so that the Center for Health Care Strategies could deploy its resources flexibly to allow the program to adapt to changing circumstances.

Since 1995, the Foundation has authorized $45 million for the Center's activities, and the Center has awarded over 100 grants to states, managed care organizations, consumer groups, and researchers.

Among the grants are awards to ten states to develop and test chronic care models. The program has given Rhode Island a grant to develop, implement, and evaluate innovative care models for children with special needs. It also has helped create a Center of Excellence for AIDS Care, which works throughout Tennessee to help providers treat Medicaid patients.

The Foundation recently reauthorized the Medicaid Managed Care program for another five years. Some of the funds will be directed to projects to help make state officials overseeing managed care programs more savvy purchasers; to strengthen the capacity of staff members of managed care organizations to organize and deliver quality managed care services to Medicaid recipients; and to help low-income consumers navigate the managed care system and become more involved in the design and monitoring of Medicaid managed care.

⎯ Research on Risk Adjustment

Individuals with chronic conditions absorb a disproportionate amount of the cost of medical care. Managed care plans have a strong financial incentive not to enroll chronically ill people whose care can cost them large amounts of money. It is easier for managed care plans to do better financially by avoiding risk than by utilizing practices that improve quality of care, and some studies indicate that they may attract and enroll healthier populations. Experts say that developing a method to pay plans for the extra resources it takes to care for patients with expensive, resource-intensive conditions—a risk adjustment mechanism—is critical for realizing the theoretical potential of managed care to save costs and increase quality. In fact, finding a risk adjustment mechanism is considered by some to be the Holy Grail of health care financing in a prepaid era.

In addition to a number of related research projects funded under the Changes in Health Care Financing and Organization program, the Foundation, in 1997, awarded $2.4 million to the University of California at San Francisco's Institute for Health Policy Studies to assess the accuracy of current risk identification methods and lay the foundation for a risk adjustment mechanism that will compensate health plans for accepting chronically ill people. Harold Luft, who is directing the project, says risk adjustment methods attempt to counteract the financial incentives placed on health plans and providers that foster disenrolling and/or limiting treatment to patients with chronic conditions. In a risk adjusted system, plans and providers are paid for the risk they assume in treating patients with high-cost conditions. Through incremental increases in payments for specific disease and conditions, he says, payments should also motivate plans and providers to track and efficiently treat chronically ill people.

Experts say that such initiatives are critical for the future of health plans to care for their sickest enrollees and compete for sick patients. "I have heard health plans say, 'We have an absolutely outstanding AIDS clinic, but we don't want to talk about it because we don't want to attract more people with AIDS.' If there is an applicable risk adjuster, plans will see that being a magnet is a way to be profitable," Luft says.

—— Gauging Managed Care's Impact on Health Systems Change

With prospects for wholesale health care reform dimming, the United States adopted a de-facto policy in 1994 emphasizing the role of the private market and competition in health care. At that time, staff members felt that The Robert Wood Johnson Foundation should establish an entity that would produce unbiased analysis and credible information about the effect of competition and managed care on access to health care, as well as its quality and cost, and that would communicate the findings to interested parties and the public at large. In 1994, the Foundation authorized funds to establish the Center for Studying Health System Change. It essentially was trying to understand, and build public knowledge about, whether the changes under way in the health system were resulting in better or worse care for Americans.

In debating alternative designs for a tracking initiative, staff members considered the challenge that, like politics, all health care is local. National surveys and studies, while comprehensive, lose the texture of local change and can miss significant trends. On the other hand, purely local or market analysis cannot determine what factors can be generalized and which are idiosyncratic to a particular community. The staff concluded that the proper approach would track market changes and their impact on people at the community level but also to engineer the sampling strategy so that national lessons could be learned.

Using this framework, the Center set up a community tracking study to follow how health care is organized and delivered in different communities. The study involves surveys of households, physicians, and employers. The Center surveys 60 communities every two years and 12 of those are studied in depth. One of the chief goals of the tracking project is to place findings about local change within a national context and show how managed care really responds to the different community markets and niches it operates in.

Although this kind of initiative requires a long-term perspective to gauge its impact, the Foundation has put a lot of weight behind it. Since 1995, it has authorized $104.7 million for Center and related activities.

Through routine briefings, forums, and published papers, the Center releases information gathered through its research to policymakers and the media. One of its earliest contributions was to dispel the myth, prevalent in the 1990s, that communities would follow a fairly linear path, from low managed care penetration to high, with progressive consolidation of health care systems. Paul Ginsburg, a health economist who directs the Center, says, "We've shown through our work that no one city is a barometer and that the paths they are taking are quite different."

In 1997, the Center held a briefing on Wall Street revealing that the profits HMOs had been making were on the wane. This briefing, covered heavily by the national press, belied the notion that HMOs were flush with money. It provided a better sense of the volatility of the private insurance market. "A lot of useful information has been shared through these Wall Street meetings," Ginsburg says. "The Washington policy makers and the Washington health policy media were not in touch with the Wall Street experts, who really have a useful perspective to bring to the debate."

In early 1998, the Center also released a major study on the effect of managed care on the provision of charity or unreimbursed care. The study pointed out that doctors who earn most of their income from HMOs or managed care plans devote less time to charity care than other physicians. That study also found that charity care was less available in communities where managed care is more prevalent than in places where it hasn't taken root as strongly.[15]

Initially, Foundation leaders were worried that the Center might be viewed as pushing a particular agenda, but so far that doesn't seem to be true. The challenge remains, however, how to get the information gathered from the Center's research into the consciousness of policymakers, the media, and the public. The task for the Foundation and the research community, observers say, is to move beyond the traditional academic audience to the community at large.

⸺ Managed Care and Behavioral Health

Nearly half of the nation's premature deaths and 70 percent of health care costs are directly linked to unhealthy behavior, including tobacco use and substance abuse. Studies have shown that changing behavior not only can improve health but also has the potential to curb health spending on preventable diseases. Because managed care plans can take a population perspective, they provide a potential platform for supporting population approaches to behavior change to improve health. Thus, beginning in the mid-1990s, the Foundation has begun to test the use of managed care as a vehicle to promote healthy lifestyles. In the tobacco arena, for example, the Foundation was able to harvest the fruits from its earlier investments in the National Committee for Quality Assurance.

In 1996, the Agency for Health Care Policy and Research, or AHCPR, issued smoking cessation guidelines to help providers and HMOs identify and treat their patients who use tobacco and to deliver antismoking messages to those who do not. The Foundation worked with a number of health and antitobacco organizations to suggest that the NCQA incorporate the guidelines into its HEDIS 2000 health plan report cards. This effort succeeded. Plans seeking accreditation are now required to measure and report the percentage of enrollees who are current smokers or quitters as well as the proportion of those who received advice to quit smoking from their doctor.

To help plans implement the AHCPR guidelines and prepare for the new HEDIS measure, the Foundation in 1996 developed a program called Addressing Tobacco in Managed Care. It is providing up to $5.3 million in grants for assessing projects designed to reduce rates of tobacco use among managed care enrollees. The four-year program is under the joint direction of the University of Wisconsin-Madison's Michael Fiore and Susan Curry of the Group Health Cooperative of Puget Sound. Fiore says that the project's objective is to identify tobacco cessation initiatives that can be integrated into a wide variety of health plans. Through this process, he says, "we hope to make it easier for managed care organizations to help their patients quit tobacco use."

In a similar fashion, the Foundation is trying to disseminate effective approaches to reducing excessive alcohol consumption. Most problem drinkers are not alcoholics, but they drink excessively or in a way that raises significant risks, such as drinking and driving. Screening and brief intervention, or SBI, approaches have been found effective in primary care settings, and managed care provides a potentially promising venue for diffusing this approach. To promote this idea, the Foundation is working with the Foundation for Accountability, based in Portland, Oregon, on a project to find a way to get providers to adopt SBI approaches among managed care enrollees.

—— Reflections—Managed Care and the Foundation

Despite managed care's hold on health care policy and delivery, its future is far from secure. The industry has a tarnished reputation, the easy profitability of the early 1990s has disappeared, and consolidation is occurring throughout the country. Some of the oldest, most mature health plans, such as Kaiser, have suffered major fiscal losses. Others, such as Harvard Pilgrim Health Care, were placed in state receivership. Managed care leaders are fighting battles in statehouses and in Congress over various patient's "bill of rights" measures and whether consumers should have the right to sue HMOs. Even the product liability lawyers have gotten into the act, attempting to apply legal strategies similar to those which worked on the tobacco industry.

Some policy analysts have predicted the end of managed care, but this seems unlikely, since no new, superior species of organization has emerged. The nation continues to spend more than a trillion dollars a year on health care, with population health indices far from the top compared with those of other industrialized nations. Over 44 million Americans now lack health insurance, and health care costs, while moderating throughout the latter 1990s, are starting to creep upward again, driven by scientific advances, new technology, and an aging population. Managed care is inextricably linked to these fundamental health policy debates.

Over the years, the Foundation's work in managed care has evolved as a parallel to the industry's development. In the early years, The Robert Wood Johnson Foundation sought to expand nonprofit prepaid group practice, a strategy that was redirected when the limits to its growth became clear. By investing more heavily in expanding nonprofit HMOs, would the Foundation have altered the industry's evolution? It's highly doubtful. Philanthropic activity can accelerate and catalyze action. But rarely can it move a field in a dynamic environment that is affected by a slew of uncontrollable factors. The conditions that promoted the growth of for-profit HMOs provided such a fertile soil that their initial success was inevitable.

In the 1980s and 1990s, the Foundation emphasized better under-standing of managed care, tracking market change, and focusing on particular domains of managed care. In retrospect, these efforts, while providing useful information and experience, could have better antic-ipated the major policy issues now arising. The Foundation learned that supporting innovation in a rapidly changing environment requires a flexible "action research" approach rather than static exper-imental designs.

Another area in which the Foundation could have been more active is in helping develop managed care leaders. One could argue that phil-anthropic support is unnecessary for the development of leadership in the private business sector. On the other hand, many other foun-dations, such as Sloan and Kauffman, have developed effective lead-ership programs with industry. The managed care industry is facing enormous and complex challenges. Foundation backing of leadership development initiatives in this area could have provided more human capital able to offer creative solutions.

Finally, the Foundation has consistently been accused by a variety of parties of being for or against managed care. Its contributions reveal that it is neither. The Foundation supports efforts that improve health and health care access for the American people. Managed care, what-ever shape it takes in the future, will be an important part of achiev-ing those objectives.

Notes

1. Personal communication, public affairs offices at the American Association of Health Plans and the Health Care Financing Administration, November, 1999.
2. Interstudy Fact Sheets dated June 1985 and November 1985.
3. Interstudy Fact Sheet dated June 1985.
4. P. Starr. *The Social Transformation of American Medicine*. New York: Basic Books, 1982, p. 396.
5. Ibid.
6. Interstudy Fact Sheet dated June 1985.
7. G. Anders, *Health Against Wealth: HMOs and the Breakdown of Medical Trust* (Boston: Houghton Mifflin, 1996), page 231.
8. R. H. Miller and H. S. Luft. "Managed Care Plan Performance Since 1980: A Literature Analysis." *The Journal of the American Medical Association*, 1994, *271*(19), 1512–1519.

9. *Chicago Tribune*, 2/12/1996.

10. K. A. Phillips et al. "Use of Preventive Services by Managed Care Enrollees: An Updated Perspective." *Health Affairs*, 2000, *19*(1), 102–116.

11. Interstudy Fact Sheet dated July 1991.

12. This initiative is discussed in L. Lopez. "Providing Care—Not Cure—for Patients with Chronic Conditions." In S. Isaacs and J. Knickman, (eds.), *To Improve Health and Health Care 1998–1999: The Robert Wood Johnson Foundation Anthology.* San Francisco: Jossey-Bass, 1998.

13. HCFA Office of Managed Care. *Medicaid Managed Care Enrollment Report, Summary Statistics, June 1995* and HCFA Press Office, personal communication, May, 2000.

14. HCFA Medicaid Bureau. *Medicaid Coordinated Care Enrollment Report: Summary Statistics as of June 30, 1992.*

15. P. J. Cunningham et al. "Managed Care and Physicians' Provision of Charity Care." *The Journal of the American Medical Association*, 1999, *281*(12), 1087–1092.

CHAPTER FIVE

⟿ Integrating Acute and Long-Term Care for the Elderly

Joseph Alper and Rosemary Gibson

Editors' Introduction

One of the principles that help explain the logic—or lack of logic—in the health care system is this: financing drives the organization of services. This principle is especially important for frail or physically disabled people who depend largely on government to finance their health care. Two distinct financing—and, therefore, delivery—systems that do not coordinate with each other have developed: the first system, Medicare, the federal government program for people over 65 and severely disabled individuals, pays for acute medical care. Except for stays immediately following hospitalization, it does not pay for nursing home care; nor does it cover supportive services, such as help in cleaning and cooking. The second system, Medicaid, a federal and state program for poor people, does pay for nursing home care and, in some states, supportive services. The two systems are cumbersome and difficult to navigate, particularly for poor, elderly people who are eligible for both Medicare and Medicaid.

A challenge for those trying to improve the care of poor older people is making the financing and delivery of services more rational and understandable. The challenge has been picked up by The Robert Wood Johnson Foundation, whose interest flows naturally from one of its three goals: to improve care and support for people with chronic health conditions. The Foundation's grant making has focused on improving acute, chronic, and supportive care for people with chronic conditions. However, improvements can happen only when financial incentives for providers are changed and when new models of organizing care emerge.

This chapter by Joseph Alper and Rosemary Gibson chronicles the Foundation's efforts to develop and support programs that integrate the financing and delivery of long-term care services for poor elderly and disabled people. The Foundation's grantees have devised strategies—many of them based on managed care—from which a number of creative models have emerged. But many older people, when given a choice, have rejected managed care approaches and the loss of independence they imply. The goal of developing coordinated services accessible to the majority of those with disabling conditions remains unmet.

Joseph Alper is a free-lance writer specializing in health care. He contributed a chapter to last year's *Anthology* on assisted living for elderly people. Rosemary Gibson, a senior program officer at The Robert Wood Johnson Foundation, has played a key role in the Foundation's chronic care grant making. She took the lead in designing a national program to improve services for the developmentally disabled, and has developed a set of national programs to improve the quality of care for terminally ill people.

At the start of the twenty-first century, many Americans face difficulties in trying to get the best care from a fragmented health care system that is often hard to navigate. This is particularly true for people with multiple chronic conditions that require them to see different physicians and other health care professionals in geographically dispersed settings. The challenge is especially burdensome for the nation's elderly, since they bear a disproportionate number of chronic conditions.

But as big a problem as this is today, it is poised to become far worse. With the aging of the American population, the need for medical care in all its forms—acute and long-term—is set to rise dramatically. With that rise, the health care system is bound to become even more difficult to navigate, particularly for the frail elderly.

Integrating Health Care for Poor Seniors

Why is the health care system in the United States so difficult to navigate? One reason is that for the most part, the nation's acute and long-term care systems function separately, with little integration between them. Acute care is provided by physicians in hospitals and doctors' offices; its chief aim is to diagnose and treat medical conditions and to perform periodic activities to maintain health and prevent illness. For the nation's elderly, most acute care involves managing episodic flare-ups of problems related to long-term chronic conditions such as heart disease and diabetes.

Long-term care is assistance given over a sustained period to people who have long-term difficulties in functioning because of a chronic condition or disability. Long-term care can be community-based—in the home or in an adult day services program, for instance—or it can be in an institutional setting such as a nursing home or an assisted-living facility. Provided mainly by nurses and nurses' aides, it consists of two elements: management of chronic conditions and supportive (or custodial) services such as assistance with bathing, dressing, and cooking.

Ideally, acute and long-term care systems should work together to ensure that a patient's entire health and daily living needs are met. Nursing home residents are likely to have more severe chronic illnesses than other older persons. This is all the more reason they need care to manage their existing chronic conditions and to prevent new ones. Yet many nursing home residents do not get the kind of care that promotes good health and looks after their chronic conditions. As a result, they are often sent to hospital emergency rooms for treatment of an acute illness that might otherwise have been avoided by better management of an underlying chronic condition.

An important reason that acute and long-term care are not effectively integrated is that these services often are paid for by different government programs, each of which has its own purposes and rules. Medicare provides health insurance coverage for people 65 and older and for those with long-term disabilities, irrespective of income. Administered by the federal government, it covers acute medical services, especially physician and hospital care. Nursing home care is available only for a limited duration for patients who need skilled care after having been hospitalized—recovering from a hip fracture, for example. Medicare does not cover nursing home care for elderly people whose primary needs are custodial—those, for example, who require help with daily activities such as bathing and meal preparation. Similarly, although Medicare's home health coverage was expanded in 1990, it is still relatively limited. In short, Medicare is not an insurance program for those who need long-term care.

In contrast, Medicaid is a state-administered program, funded jointly by the federal government and the states, that provides health insurance coverage for the poor. Medicaid pays for physician's services and hospital care and, in addition, covers the cost of nursing home care, including custodial care, for low-income seniors. In many states, Medicaid funds some community-based care.

Although integration of acute and long-term care services is important for *all* seniors, there is a subset—poor elderly people—who could benefit from making both the delivery and the financing of acute and long-term care more rational. They are the so-called "dual eligibles" who qualify for Medicare because they are over age 65 and for Medicaid because of their low income. Dual-eligible seniors often have complex chronic care needs. They often need long-term care— both to manage their chronic conditions and to provide supportive services—and have frequent contact with the acute care system.

In 1997, the number of dual-eligible seniors was estimated to be 6.7 million—they constituted 17 percent of all Medicare beneficiaries but absorbed 28 percent of Medicare expenditures.[1] Dual-eligible beneficiaries use more Medicare services across the board—hospital, skilled nursing facility, and home health care. Of these dual eligibles, 33 percent use emergency rooms in a given year, compared with 18 percent of Medicare-only beneficiaries. On the Medicaid side, dual eligibles represented 19 percent of all beneficiaries in 1997 but accounted for 35 percent of all spending.[2]

The Health Care Financing Administration, or HFCA, which oversees both the Medicare and Medicaid programs, has allowed states to develop projects to explore new ways of integrating Medicare's acute benefits with Medicaid's long-term care benefits to provide a more seamless system of care. HCFA does not provide startup funds for the projects, but does enable them to bill Medicare and Medicaid for the services they provide.

What would an integrated system of care mean for frail elderly people? Integration means that multiple systems act and feel as a seamless one.[3] For those residing in nursing homes, integration means having good skin care to prevent bedsores and good primary care to prevent pneumonia from developing among the most frail group of elderly patients. For seniors living in the community, integrated care might mean a physician arranging for a home visit from a social worker to identify and address risk factors that could cause a fall and a broken hip.

Since the early 1980s, The Robert Wood Johnson Foundation has nurtured projects aimed at integrating acute and long-term care. One of the first of those, the Program of All-inclusive Care for the Elderly, or PACE, is an attempt to develop models of a seamless service delivery system for very frail seniors.

—— An Early Model: The Program of All-Inclusive Care for the Elderly

A fully integrated model of acute and long-term care was developed by On Lok Senior Health Services in San Francisco in the late 1970s. By 1983, On Lok's model had become a federal demonstration project, and this status allowed it to receive financing from Medicare and Medicaid that was placed in a single pool. To build on the On Lok model, in 1988, The Robert Wood Johnson Foundation provided $5.8 million for the Program of All-Inclusive Care for the Elderly. The four-year program supported the replication of the On-Lok model of integrated care for poor seniors at six sites (Boston, Massachusetts; the

Bronx, New York; Columbia, South Carolina; El Paso, Texas; Milwaukee, Wisconsin; and Portland, Oregon).

The PACE model is characterized by a focus on the significantly impaired frail elderly; a team-managed approach to care that integrates a comprehensive package of acute and long-term health services in both inpatient and outpatient settings; and capitated, or fixed-rate per patient, financing from both Medicare and Medicaid. Like On Lok, PACE provides a viable alternative to nursing home care for very frail seniors.

To enroll in PACE, a person must be 55 or older, need nursing home care based on the state's standards, and reside at home in the program's defined geographic area. An interdisciplinary team based at the local PACE Center, which also provides adult day care, orchestrates all care. Though enrollees receive routine care at the PACE Center or at home, specialty and inpatient care are readily available whenever needed.

"What we've done with PACE is to completely integrate services and financing for both acute and long-term care, and by doing so we've created a fully integrated managed care system for the frail elderly," says Jennie Chin Hansen, On Lok's executive director and a PACE board member. "Our overall goal, which I think PACE achieves, is to maximize each enrollee's autonomy and continued community residence and, at the same time, provide quality care at lower cost to Medicare and Medicaid."

Hansen explains that under terms negotiated with HCFA, a PACE Center receives monthly capitation payments from Medicare and Medicaid, as well as payments from individuals who are financially ineligible for Medicaid and who pay that portion of the monthly fee themselves. Medicare bases its payment on a methodology, developed to reimburse Medicare health maintenance organizations, or HMOs, that accounts for regional disparities in the cost of medical care and that is then adjusted to reflect the frailty of PACE enrollees compared to the average Medicare beneficiary. In 1998, the monthly Medicare capitation payment to PACE programs ranged from $877 to $1,775. PACE Medicaid payments are based on state-specific estimates of the fee-for-service costs for comparable long-term-care populations. In 1998, Medicaid monthly capitation rates ranged from $1,750 to $4,301.

"One key to the PACE model is that all payments are pooled by the PACE site and used for any program-eligible senior without regard to traditional restrictions, giving the site greater flexibility to deliver whatever services are needed," Hansen says. The allocation of those services, she explains, is determined through continual assessments of each patient's needs by the interdisciplinary team of primary care physician, nurse, social worker, rehabilitation therapist, home health workers, and others.

In the Balanced Budget Act of 1997, Congress authorized PACE to graduate from a federal demonstration program to a permanently approved Medicare provider, joining the ranks of the thousands of other accepted providers that receive regular payments from Medicare. In addition, the Balanced Budget Act made PACE a state option under the Medicaid regulations—each state can now add local PACE program to its list of permanent regular providers. The Act also increased the authorized number of PACE sites nationwide from 15 in 1997 to 40 in 1998, with an additional 20 added to this cap each year thereafter, enabling a systematic expansion of the model. Finally, the Act also allowed for up to 10 sites to be run by for-profit entities. This step of making PACE a permanent Medicare and Medicaid provider was based on these considerations:

- Despite PACE enrollees' level of frailty, their rate of hospital use is lower than that of the Medicare 65-plus population, which includes healthy older persons—in 1997, 2,080 days per 1,000 PACE enrollees vs. 2,158 days per 1,000 Medicare beneficiaries.[4]
- PACE enrollees have shorter lengths of stay in the hospital than the over-65 Medicare population as a whole—4.1 vs. 6.6 days.[5]
- Medicare's rate-setting methodology for PACE guarantees a minimum 5 percent savings. However, several studies suggest substantially higher savings from PACE. A study commissioned by HCFA reported Medicare savings of 38 percent in the first six months after enrollment and 16 percent savings over the next six months.[6]
- PACE offers policy makers a less costly community-based alternative to constructing new nursing home beds.[7]

In preparation for the growth spurred by the 1997 Balanced Budget Act, the National PACE Association, with funding from The Robert Wood Johnson Foundation, completed the development of standards and an accreditation review process in 1997. The National

PACE Association is now conducting a pilot study, in collaboration with an accrediting body, to test the standards and make necessary modifications in preparation for formal accreditation. The accreditation process is a way to ensure that new PACE programs will remain faithful to the original PACE model.

As of February, 2000, about 6,000 frail seniors were enrolled at twenty-five PACE sites around the country, reflecting the growth of the program. Enrollment in PACE is modest in relation to the number of frail elderly who could benefit from integrated acute and long-term care. But the significance of PACE on health care for the elderly is larger than its numerical impact might imply. In the 1980s, before it became a government-approved demonstration site, PACE developed as a neighborhood program and not as a large-scale health plan. At the time, before the involvement of The Robert Wood Johnson Foundation, start-up capital was scarce, yet the program was still able to build itself into a working model. The principles of managed care and managing risk were being tried and tested, and there was little, if any, experience in the country in managing all the health care and supportive service needs of the frail elderly under a capitation payment. PACE tackled each of these problems.

The challenge that remains is to take the integration of acute and long-term care to scale. Because of its reliance on the PACE Center, an adult day services facility of sorts, the program may not work well in sparsely populated rural areas. And PACE, as it currently exists, is designed to treat groups of less than 200 adults. More and larger efforts are needed.

—— The Minnesota Senior Health Options Program

Minnesota Senior Health Options is an attempt to expand significantly the integration of services for frail elders who are eligible for both Medicare and Medicaid. With the help of a Foundation grant, Minnesota became the first state to receive approval from HCFA for a statewide program to integrate acute and long-term care with funding from both Medicare and Medicaid. A program that has the potential to serve all dual eligibles in a state makes it possible to reach many more frail seniors, in contrast to demonstration projects at a single or only a few sites.

In 1997, Minnesota Senior Health Options, a five-year demonstration project, began enrolling its first participants in the seven-county metropolitan Minneapolis-St. Paul area. The central feature of the program is its reliance on Minnesota's extensive network of managed care providers and the fact that HMOs have a long history in the state and are widely accepted as providers of care by state residents. "That's one advantage we have here in Minnesota," says Pamela Parker, the program's director. "Minnesotans accept the role of managed care and have had good experiences with it over a long period of time."

Minnesota has contracted with three of the Minneapolis-St. Paul metropolitan area's five largest health plans to provide all Medicare and Medicaid services, including home and community-based services and 180 days of nursing home care. If a frail senior needs more than 180 days of care in a nursing home, the nursing home is reimbursed on a fee-for-service basis. Since 77 percent of enrollees reside in a nursing home, nursing home care is an important part of Minnesota Senior Health Options.

The program's home and community-based services include case management, companion services, caregiver training, extended home health aide, extended personal care assistance, adult foster care, adult day care, assisted living, residential services, homemaker services, home delivered meals, respite care, home modification, and supplies and equipment. Each senior has a "care coordinator" to assist with care planning and service access.

As of January 2000, enrollment in the program stood at 3,420, or about 25 percent of the dual-eligible population in the seven-county metropolitan area. Thirty-eight percent of enrollees are over age 85. In a survey conducted at that time, half of the Options program enrollees noticed a marked improvement in services when they enrolled, and 70 percent said their transition to the new program was smooth. "To me, it was like a gift from God," said Mae, a sunny woman in her mid-60s who participates in Senior Options. Another enrollee, Marge, said, "Now I see a doctor every six months, and if I don't call to make an appointment, someone calls me. I think that's good." For Sarah, who couldn't get any services before enrolling in the Minnesota program, the program has been a lifesaver: "They take very good care of me now. My coordinator makes sure I get the care I need when I need it," And for Ralph, "It has given me peace of mind. I think that's what it boils down to. I didn't know what would happen to me. This was a gift."

"Overall, we feel that we've been pretty successful so far, and it's been pretty smooth running on a day-to-day basis," Parker says. "The place where we are disappointed is in how far we've been able to take the program. We've pushed the marketplace forward toward being more focused on the elderly, but reimbursement issues and fear of risk under a capitated payment system have kept two of the state's big plans from joining the program. We're trying to work with HCFA to solve that, but for now it's a sticking point."

⎯ The Medicare-Medicaid Integration National Program

Building on the experience of Minnesota Senior Health Options, in 1996 The Robert Wood Johnson Foundation established the Medicare-Medicaid Integration Program, an $8 million grant initiative. Under this program, seven states and one regional organization have received grants up to $300,000 to test ways to integrate acute and long-term care. To date, the Foundation has awarded grants to Colorado, Florida, New York, Oregon, Texas, Virginia, Washington, and the New England Consortium (Connecticut, Maine, Massachusetts, New Hampshire, Rhode Island, and Vermont). Each grantee is trying a different approach to integrating acute and long-term care, depending on the target population—urban or rural, for example. And though many of the states have found it difficult to develop a program and are only in the early stages of doing so, states such as Texas have been more successful in enrolling seniors. "It's been a trying experience for many states, and each has had to find its way, but we are seeing results now and we're starting to learn some important lessons," say Mark Meiners, the national program director at the University of Maryland Center on Aging. The Texas STAR+PLUS project and the Colorado Integrated Care and Financing Project are two examples of efforts funded under the Medicare-Medicaid Integration Program.

Texas STAR+PLUS

The Texas project, STAR+PLUS has big ambitions. The entire Medicaid population that needs acute and long-term care in Harris County, which includes Houston, is the target group for this pilot. In January, 1998, participation in STAR+PLUS became mandatory for some 55,000 Harris County residents. Half of these 55,000 residents are over age 65 and also eligible for Medicare; the others are under age 65 and eligible for Medicaid only. STAR+PLUS is different from the other projects, since it integrates acute and long-term care only under Medicaid. It doesn't address the integration of Medicare financing or delivery systems.

STAR+PLUS contracts with three HMOs, which are responsible for providing acute and long-term care, including nursing home care and expanded home and community-based services. "We felt that this gives the HMOs an incentive to provide innovative, cost-effective care from the outset in order to prevent or delay the need for more costly institutionalization," says Pamela Coleman, director of STAR+PLUS. HMOs are required to conduct a health assessment for each new enrollee within 30 days of enrollment. For the 1,500 nursing home residents who are enrolled, the nursing home staff provides the care in the nursing homes and the HMOs make monthly visits to check up on them.

In addition, the state requires the HMOs to provide each enrollee with a care coordinator who is responsible for ensuring that the patient receives integrated acute and long-term care. Care coordinators make home visits and identify unmet needs, some of which are not the usual long-term care needs but are nonetheless important. For example, some care coordinators authorize pest control in unhealthy home environments and others install smoke alarms.

The main challenge has been the less-than-enthusiastic response from long-term care providers. "This has been a wakeup call for them," Coleman says. With a low nursing home occupancy rate of 81 percent, the nursing homes seem worried that the community services being offered under the program might reduce the number of people requiring institutional care. The rates paid to the nursing homes are the same for now, but the HMOs that pay the nursing homes might change the methodology for determining the rates in the future.

The picture for STAR+PLUS in Texas over the long run is uncertain. State legislators placed a moratorium on any expansion of Medicaid managed care programs in the state. STAR+PLUS has gotten caught up in this moratorium.

Colorado's Integrated Care and Financing Project

Colorado's Integrated Care and Financing Project was developed as a pilot project to integrate Medicare and Medicaid financing for dual-eligible residents of Mesa County, a largely rural county in western Colorado. Rocky Mountain HMO, which has a long history of providing managed acute health care in the county's largest city, Grand Junction, was to work with Mesa County Options for Long-Term Care, part of the Department of Human Services, to provide integrated acute and long-term care for the target population.

As the first step in this demonstration, the Colorado Department of Health Care Policy and Financing applied for approval from HCFA in September, 1995, to integrate Medicare and Medicaid financing. Two years later, HCFA granted approval to the state to go ahead, but a stumbling block emerged—HCFA and the state were unable to agree on the amount of the Medicare capitation payment that HCFA should pay to the HMO. After a series of negotiations, Colorado decided to have the Medicare contract with the HMO stay as is and providers would be paid on a fee-for-service service basis. The experience illustrates some of the difficulty in agreeing on how much health plans should be paid to care for the dually eligible population.

While the state was working intensely with HCFA to get the Medicare financing ironed out, Rocky Mountain HMO withdrew from the program because of an unrelated issue resulting from internal operating changes within the HMO. Colorado will now attempt to develop a demonstration program in Denver under the Medicare-Medicaid Integration Program.

—— The Wisconsin Partnership Program

The Wisconsin Partnership Program, funded under a different Foundation-funded national program—Building Health Systems for People With Chronic Illness—represents yet another approach to integrating acute and long-term care. Like the PACE model, the Wisconsin Partnership uses an interdisciplinary team of a physician, a nurse, a nurse practitioner, daily living assistants, and a social worker or an independent living coordinator. The teams provide acute and long-term health care for seniors eligible for both Medicare and Medicaid in four demonstration communities around the state. In contrast to PACE, where enrollees are required to use the primary care physician from the PACE team, enrollees in the Wisconsin Partnership Program can choose a primary care physician from a network of participating physicians.

One of the sites, the Community Health Partnership of Eau Claire in east central Wisconsin is particularly interesting because it serves a mostly rural population of 180,000, spread across three counties encompassing 2,500 square miles; the only major city in the area, Eau Claire, has 12,000 residents. In contrast, Milwaukee (site of another of the state's demonstrations) contains just over 960,000 people within its 241-square-mile area. "We knew it would be a challenge to serve such a sparsely populated area," says Steve Landkamer, project manger of the Wisconsin Partnership Program. "But we also knew that with the large number of dual-eligible seniors living in rural Wisconsin we were going to have to face this problem eventually. So why not do it now, before we get steamrollered by the coming wave of baby boomers reaching retirement age?"

The job of setting up the Eau Claire site fell to Karen Hodgson, chief executive officer of Community Health Partnership. "We cheated a little in getting started by focusing our initial efforts on the area within a 25-mile radius of Eau Claire," Hodgson says. "But that way, we were able to get up to speed without stretching ourselves too thin."

The 187 seniors who were enrolled as of February, 2000, have "very high levels of health care needs, the frailest of our citizens," according to Hodgson. When someone enrolls in the program, the team identifies any immediate health care needs and addresses them. The medical director at Community Health Partners, Mark Deyo-Svendsen, notes, "About 25 percent of members meet diagnostic criteria for depression." This means that there is a lot of upfront work to deal with health care needs that have been neglected, often for a long time.

After that initial assessment, the team's focus turns to prevention, an approach that appears to be working, both for the seniors enrolled in the program and for Community Health Partnership's bottom line. The project staff notes that over the three years that the program has been operating, participants are spending fewer days in the hospital and the nursing home compared to the time before they joined the program. Meanwhile, visits to the primary care physician have increased, reflecting the emphasis on prevention. "At first, we were spending heavily on physician visits to get our seniors onto the prevention track, but that spending has paid off and we now expect to be running a surplus on our budget," Deyo-Svendsen says.

A key feature of the Eau Claire project is the emphasis on in-home prevention, with social workers making home visits at least once a month, and sometimes weekly. While in the home, the social worker can spot a senior who is struggling with alcoholism, which might be hindering management of the patient's diabetes. The social worker can arrange for community resources to help the elderly person cope with the addiction.

The daily living assistants who are members of the interdisciplinary team are, in essence, the first-line care providers. Some are certified as nursing assistants who provide personal care such as dressing, feeding, and toileting. Some daily living assistants help around the house with cleaning and grocery shopping. One of the biggest challenges in the program, is "finding people who are willing to work for $7 an hour and show up for work every day," according to Hodgson. "We really count on them, and most of them do this work because they love the people they are caring for."

Team members work hard to instill a sense of responsibility so that the seniors themselves ask for and receive the appropriate amount of care. "We let our members know that although they have access to more services than they were used to, this isn't a blank check to give everyone everything that they wanted," Hodgson says. This tough message evidently sits well with members—only four people have left the program in more than three years. "Sure, people grumble sometimes, but the bottom line is that they are healthier and they are getting far more care than they used to get under the old fragmented system."

⁓ Lessons Learned

Rationalizing fragmented and unresponsive health care delivery systems is a worthy but difficult endeavor. The number of people benefiting from integrated acute and long-term care is modest in relation to the millions of elderly people who have to fend for themselves in the fragmented health care systems that are the norm in this country. The PACE model has shown that it is possible to create a seamless system of care for a very vulnerable population of frail elders. PACE programs work well because they are small, and because dedicated professionals work together to create their own system of care to meet the needs of patients. In fact, the team approach is likely to be a key factor in making integration of acute and long-term care work. It can lead to better communication among multiple providers caring for the same person and to a more consistent strategy for caring for the patient.

In contrast to the team approach is an approach that simply tries to coordinate the care offered by the long-term and acute systems.

While the team approach involves restructuring the system of delivering services, the coordination approach merely patches some of the holes in it. Nevertheless, since health care delivery systems are unlikely to undergo a major reconfiguration any time soon, coordination may be the most viable strategy to improve care on a large scale within the existing fragmented system. Care coordination will still have to juggle the opposing cultures of acute care—which exists to cure, treat, and sometimes prevent illness—and long-term care—which exists to make life better for people when there is no cure.

The Medicare-Medicaid Integration Program has stressed the importance of integrated financing between Medicare and Medicaid as key to making delivery systems work better on the ground. But making the financing of acute and long-term care more rational has proven to be challenging. It is, after all, an ambitious undertaking to get the nation's two major health care insurance programs, Medicare and Medicaid, to provide seamless financing. Yet integrated financing is not a panacea, and certainly it will not make much of a difference if integrated delivery systems are not in place. The original On Lok model of delivering services, which was replicated by PACE, grew from the ground up in San Francisco, based on what frail elders and their families needed. Then the integrated financing from Medicare and Medicaid was put in place to support the model. And while it is often the case that reimbursement procedures shape health care delivery systems, On Lok and PACE have shown us that it is possible for the delivery system to shape how care should be reimbursed.

Some state efforts to integrate acute and long-term care seemed to give priority to melding financing streams. While this is important, it's not clear that the states had health care delivery models ready that would integrate acute and long-term care. Wisconsin appears to be a step ahead; at the same time that it was revamping financing, its demonstration sites were creating new team approaches to care for frail elders. Other states relied on HMOs, nursing homes, home care providers, and others to render care in a more coordinated way. The changes needed in each of the delivery systems, and across those systems, to integrate care are not insignificant, and it's not evident that major changes in the delivery system were, in fact, made. Perhaps the attention given to the financing preempted attention to the development of models of delivering care. Developing integrated models of care needs to be a high priority and not simply follow the financing of services.

As health care providers and states attempt to develop models, component parts of integrated acute and long-term care can be distinguished: flexible benefit packages, a broad range of providers, mechanisms for effective care integration, and financing. They can be considered the building blocks, and some lessons can be drawn from the experience to date.[8] These lessons include:

> *Flexible Benefits.* Integrated models of care need a broad range of acute and long-term care benefits. The benefit package should be flexible and responsive to people's needs.

> *Broad Range of Health Care Providers.* If a program is to include a wide range of acute and long-term care services, the delivery system should have capacity and experience beyond what is offered by traditional acute and long-term care providers. Community-based long-term care, case management, and a variety of specialty providers should be part of the delivery system.

> *Care Integration.* Integrated systems need ways to assure that the broad range of health care providers work together toward the same goals for the patient. Interdisciplinary care teams and centralized member records are key elements of integrated care. Without these elements, patients will simply have a fragmented array of services under an ineffective program umbrella.

> *Integrated Financing.* Medicare and Medicaid funding should be flexible, and the incentives created by the two major payors should be aligned to eliminate cost shifting between the two programs. PACE, for example, eliminates this by pooling all capitated payments into one central fund for health care expenditures regardless of whether they come from Medicare or Medicaid.

States and providers are taking some steps toward integrating acute and long-term care. In theory, at least, integration does offer the opportunity for improvement in health outcomes. But whether such outcomes will actually result from integration is a question worthy of research.

Large-scale efforts to integrate Medicare and Medicaid financing are unlikely in the foreseeable future. Instead of integration of the whole range of acute and long-term care for a large segment of the frail elderly, it is more likely that bits and pieces will be integrated.

Housing, supportive services, and some medical care are being integrated in assisted living facilities. Advances in technology are making diagnostic testing—and better primary care—available while patients remain at home. These are small yet important steps that can be enormously helpful to patients and their families. While they will not reduce the fragmentation across the continuum of care, they are, at least, steps in the right direction.

Notes

1. P. Parker, testimony prepared for Congress, Minnesota Senior Health Options, 1999.
2. Ibid.
3. M. Booth, J. Fralich, P. Saucier, R. Mollica, and T. Riley. *Integration of Acute and Long-Term Care for Dually Eligible Beneficiaries through Managed Care.* Princeton, N.J.: The Robert Wood Johnson Foundation, August 1997.
4. A. J. White. *The Effect of PACE on Costs to Medicare.* Cambridge, Mass.: Abt Associates, 1998.
5. Ibid.
6. A. White. *Evaluation of the Program of All-inclusive Care for the Elderly (PACE) Demonstration. The Effect of PACE on Costs to Medicare: A Comparison of Medicare Capitation Rates to Projected Costs in the Absence of Pace.* Final Report to the Health Care Financing Administration. Cambridge, Mass.: Abt Associates, 1998.
7. J. C. Hansen. "Practical Lessons for Delivering Integrated Services in a Changing Environment: The PACE Model." *Generations,* Summer 1999, pp. 22–28.
8. The Muskie School of Public Service at the University of Southern Maine and the National Academy for State Health Policy. *Integration of Acute and Long-Term Care for Dually Eligible Beneficiaries through Managed Care.* Technical Assistance Paper Number 1 of the Medicare/Medicaid Integration Program. (College Park, Md.: Center on Aging at the University of Maryland, August 1997, pp. 2–3.

CHAPTER SIX

~~ The Workers' Compensation Health Initiative

At the Convergence of Work and Health

Allard E. Dembe and Jay S. Himmelstein

Editors' Introduction

In 1910, New York enacted the country's first workers' compensation law. Wisconsin followed a year later, and by 1949 every state had passed a workers' compensation statute. The theory behind workers' compensation is simple—both employees and employers trade risk for certainty. Employees exchange the risk of going to court—which could result in a financial bonanza but more likely will return nothing—for the certainty of receiving limited compensation for their work-related injuries. Employers agree to pay job-related injury claims, whether or not it was their fault, and in return are assured that they will not be sued.

Although workers' compensation was created to simplify claims and avoid lawsuits, it has evolved into an expensive, complicated, legalistic system that all-too-often pits an injured worker against an employers' insurance company In 1998, about $16 billion was paid out to provide medical care for job-related injuries and illnesses through the workers' compensation system. Although this represents just 1.3 percent of all health care spending, at its best high-quality workers' compensation care can promote the well being and employability of workers and improve the productivity of American businesses.

In the late 1980s and early 1990s, many states reformed their workers' compensation systems, allowing managed care organizations to provide medical care for injured workers and encouraging the integration of workers' compensation and other health care systems. President Clinton included similar changes as part of his health reform proposals in the early 1990s. These developments piqued the interest of The Robert Wood Johnson Foundation, which in 1995 funded a national program called the Workers' Compensation Health Initiative to better understand the workers' compensation system and to promote innovations in how care is delivered to injured workers.

This chapter by Allard Dembe and Jay Himmelstein explains the workers' compensation system, the research undertaken by the 21 grantees supported by the program, and key findings from their work. It places the findings in the context of other efforts to improve workers' compensation, and concludes with a discussion of the emerging trends and policy implications.

Allard Dembe and Jay Himmelstein are the deputy director and the director, respectively, of the Workers' Compensation Health Initiative. Both are faculty members at the University of Massachusetts Medical School in the Department of Family and Community Medicine. Himmelstein is the assistant chancellor for health policy and directs the University's Center for Health Policy and Research.

T

he numbness and pain in Lidia Fernandez's hands began in the spring of 1996 and grew steadily worse. Like many immigrant female workers in Manhattan's garment district, Lidia had worked for years in a small, congested factory operating sewing machines, tending equipment for making button holes, and, most recently, as a "floor girl" involved in inspecting wedding gowns, clipping off excess thread, and hanging the finished dresses on elevated racks. Many of Lidia's co-workers—predominantly young Italian, Chinese, and Latin American women—experienced similar hand and wrist discomfort. Her pain and numbness progressed, but Lidia kept working. "I didn't have a choice," Lidia said. "I have to continue working. I live by myself. I need the money." When the pain finally forced her to see a doctor, she was distressed to learn that her union's health insurance plan would not cover the costs of her medical care: "They said my problem is caused by my job and should be covered by workers' compensation. They wouldn't have anything to do with it." When she filed a claim with her employer for workers' compensation, she was similarly disappointed. "They denied coverage," she said. "The claims adjuster didn't believe that it was work-related." In a desperate attempt to get the matter resolved, Lidia hired a lawyer, who pursued the case through the adjudication process of the New York State Workers' Compensation Board. More than three years have now passed, and Lidia's claim is still pending. "The judge's decision is expected next month," Lidia said. "It's been a nightmare."

Unfortunately, Lidia's experience is not at all uncommon. Recent studies by investigators from the Mt. Sinai School of Medicine found that 79 percent of claims for work-related carpal tunnel syndrome in New York are denied by workers' compensation insurance carriers.[1] Of those cases adjudicated through the state's administrative justice process, more than 96 percent are eventually decided in favor of the injured worker. But the researchers found that the length of time between claim filing and the judge's decision averages 429 days. Since all work-related disorders are supposed to be covered exclusively through workers' compensation insurance, most general health plans will not pay for medical treatment once a workers' compensation claim has been filed. Consequently, injured workers are often left without access to effective medical care, despite the presumably comprehensive and full coverage guaranteed to virtually all workers under state workers' compensation laws. Similar barriers to access for medical care involving occupational conditions have been verified in numerous other studies.[2]

In one respect, Lidia was lucky. Her union, the Union of Needletrades, Industrial and Textile Employees, or UNITE, operates a special occupational clinic at the Union Health Center in New York City. With grant support from The Robert Wood Johnson Foundation's Workers' Compensation Health Initiative, UNITE has developed a financing plan that allows a worker to borrow money from the union's benefit funds to pay participating physicians while workers' compensation claims are being adjudicated. Through this plan, Lidia was eventually able to obtain diagnostic testing and therapeutic surgery for her carpal tunnel syndrome. "If it weren't for the UNITE program, I wouldn't have received any care," she said. "I would have been helpless." With continued funding from The Robert Wood Johnson Foundation, researchers from Mt. Sinai and the New School University's Center for Health Policy Research are now systematically examining the impact of the UNITE program on patients' medical and vocational outcomes and the quality of care.

Three hundred miles to the north, in Clinton County, New York, near the Canadian border, Daniel Devito remembers his encounter with the workers' compensation medical care system. Devito, a 31-year-old employee of a local bottling company, fell over a pallet while delivering cases of bottled soda. Two weeks later, his resulting backache had gotten worse, and pain appeared along the sciatic nerve in the back of his leg. "One night, the pain in my leg was so intense I couldn't sleep," he said. "By five in the morning, I couldn't move my leg and the pain was unbearable. All I could think about was getting to the emergency room. I called for an ambulance."

The ambulance brought Devito to the Champlain Valley Physicians Hospital Medical Center in Plattsburgh, 15 miles away. The area around Plattsburgh, like many rural areas in the United States, has few medical providers who specialize in occupational medicine or are well-versed in workers' compensation insurance and rehabilitation for injured workers. Clinton County has virtually no penetration by traditional health maintenance organizations or managed care service providers. The region has few of the resources needed for aggressively managing the medical treatment of work injuries. The 1995 closing of a local Air Force base had resulted in the loss of 2,500 jobs, delivering a devastating blow to the region's economy. In an attempt to revitalize the area's employment base, a local group of business and health-care leaders identified the improvement of workers' compensation medical care as a key component in attracting new industry. A community coalition was established—the North Country On the Job Network, or NCOTJN—with representatives from the Chamber of Commerce, local employers, health care providers, labor organizations, city and county government, and the Champlain Valley Physicians Hospital Medical Center.

When Devito reached the hospital, a nurse case manager from NCOTJN was there to meet him. During the next four weeks, the NCOTJN case manager stayed with Devito at every step of his treatment and recovery, making sure that he received appropriate care and was quickly referred to qualified specialists, expediting office visits, ensuring that no delays in treatment occurred, and acting as a liaison to facilitate communication and planning between the patient, his employer, the workers' compensation insurer, and a variety of health care providers. Unlike typical workers' compensation arrangements in which the case manager works directly for a compensation insurer or the employer, the NCOTJN case manger is officially an agent of the community coalition, representing the patient's and the community's interests. In the contentious world of workers' compensation medicine, which often pits employers and their insurers against workers and their lawyers, the objective perspective of the NCOTJN case manager was welcomed.

"I trusted her better than I trusted the doctors," Devito says of his case manager. When Devito twice suffered a severe allergic reaction to medication prescribed by his doctors, the NCOTJN case manager suggested that Devito discuss the situation with a local pharmacist and have the pharmacist call the doctors to work out a change of medication. "It was a brilliant idea that I wouldn't have thought of myself," he says—one of several good ideas that he credits with achieving his successful recovery. "She found a physical therapist right in my town, because I was having difficulty making the trip to Plattsburgh. She even got me hooked up with a chiropractor, which would have been almost impossible to get approved without her help."

Case management is only one of several services offered by the NCOTJN community coalition. It regularly sponsors educational seminars on occupational medicine, bringing in national experts to meet with local providers. The coalition employs a telemedicine system for consultations with providers in remote areas who are treating workers' compensation cases. Through a grant provided to NCOTJN by the Workers' Compensation Health Initiative, researchers from the Duke University School of Medicine are conducting studies to assess the impact of the coalition's efforts on the cost and the quality of care, along with the workers' experiences in getting appropriate medical treatment and attaining full recovery. For Daniel Devito, the efforts of the NCOTJN and its case manager are easy to summarize. In his opinion, "She was on my side."

⎯⎯ Obtaining Care for Work-Related Conditions

These case histories illustrate some of the many challenges individuals face in seeking treatment for work-related injuries and illnesses, and a few of the new approaches being taken to improve workers' compensation medical care. Although workers' compensation insurance was originally intended to ensure prompt access to medical care for all injured workers, significant barriers to obtaining appropriate care abound. For example, to qualify for workers' compensation coverage, a patient's condition must be clinically determined to have been caused in the workplace. In the early twentieth century, when workers' compensation laws were first enacted, most job-related cases involved acute, traumatic injuries that were relatively easy to identify and trace to workplace accidents. But the majority of today's cases involve nonspecific back pain, hand and wrist discomfort, musculoskeletal ailments, respiratory illnesses, and other disorders for which there is an indistinct connection with job activities and a range of reasonable medical opinion about the degree of work-relatedness.

Few medical schools provide extensive training in the recognition and treatment of occupational ailments. Practicing physicians have little time or incentive to visit patients' workplaces or fully investigate possible occupational causes of illness. Many clinicians dislike the adversarial nature of workers' compensation and the extensive administrative procedures required in some states when treating occupational cases. As a result, some physicians either avoid seeing injured workers altogether or fail to evaluate adequately suspected work-related conditions. A recent study by researchers from Harvard University found that physicians at a large health maintenance organization failed to diagnose properly and report cases of occupational asthma 21 percent of the time, in part because they did not obtain detailed work histories.[3]

Medical care delivered to injured workers often requires specialized services that go beyond what would be customary in the typical primary care setting. For example, to prove that a patient's condition is work-related, and thus eligible for payment through workers' compensation, special diagnostic testing may be required. Moreover, to qualify patients for the wage-replacement benefits that are also provided through workers' compensation insurance, medical providers must often perform additional tests and procedures, including the evaluation of impairment and vocational function, and the assessment of job demands and work limitations. Medical practitioners are expected to consider the patient's needs for retraining and job accommodation and to work closely with physical therapists, occupational therapists, and rehabilitation specialists to achieve a speedy recovery of vocational function and minimize work disability. These medical actions are often surrounded by controversy in the combative workers' compensation system. This can complicate the medical care delivery process and embroil all parties, including doctors, in legal actions and lengthy administrative procedures. These factors can delay, and possibly jeopardize, the provision of needed services.

Medical care for workplace injuries and illnesses is one element in the broader context of management-labor relationships. The employer generally selects the workers' compensation insurance carrier and determines medical care arrangements. In most states, employees are restricted in their ability to alter the plan or choose their own medical care providers. In many cases, injured employees are not permitted to obtain care from their regular primary care practitioner, and this restriction may result in discontinuous care and incomplete medical records. The recent introduction of managed care and restricted provider networks into the workers' compensation setting is seen by some workers as part of a concerted campaign to strengthen employer control over care and further restrict employee choice.

Indeed, in many states, managed care provisions were first introduced as part of broad workers' compensation reform legislation enacted between 1992 and 1994. This legislation aimed at curbing the escalating cost of workers' compensation medical care in the late 1980s and early 1990s. During that period, average workers' compensation medical care costs grew at an annual rate of 14 percent, exceeding by 30 percent the rise in total national health expenditures. In response, more than twenty states passed laws to contain costs. These laws contained provisions that reduced wage-loss benefits, tightened eligibility requirements, and introduced the use of restricted networks, utilization review, discounted fee schedules, and mandatory treatment guidelines. Until recently, few studies had been undertaken to assess the impact of these reforms on the costs and quality of care.

⎯⎯ Improving Workers' Compensation Medical Care

The Robert Wood Johnson Foundation's involvement in workers' compensation was sparked in 1993 when it received several proposals from state workers' compensation agencies to evaluate pilot cost-control and managed care programs. Its interest was further stimulated that same year by the Clinton administration's call for integrating workers' compensation and general health care into a single "twenty-four hour" coverage scheme under the proposed Health Security Act. In 1995, the Foundation established the Workers' Compensation Health Initiative, or WCHI, a national grant making program supporting demonstration and evaluation projects to test new models for improving quality and containing the cost of workers' compensation medical care. A national program office was created at the University of Massachusetts Medical School to direct this six-year, $6 million initiative.

In the mid-1990s, other agencies also launched efforts to study and improve health care for injured workers. In April 1996, the National Institute for Occupational Safety and Health, or NIOSH, designated occupational health services research as one of 21 priority areas in its National Occupational Research Agenda, and instituted two rounds of grant awards in 1996 and 1999 for investigators studying the delivery of medical services to workers with occupational injuries and illnesses. At about the same time, the nonprofit Workers' Compensation Research Institute, in Cambridge, Massachusetts, began a multiyear effort to create a national research database for studies of workers' compensation medical care and to conduct analyses of the impact of provider networks and other new health care developments.

Since its inception, the Workers' Compensation Health Initiative has awarded 21 grants to a variety of institutions and agencies. Projects supported through the Initiative have included 24-hour medical care plans that cover both work-related and nonoccupational cases, the creation of new techniques for managing work disability, the development and evaluation of medical practice guidelines for work-related disorders, the formation of community- and union-based coalitions to enhance workers' compensation health care, innovative approaches to case management for workplace injuries, and a nationwide effort to develop standardized performance measures for workers' compensation managed care organizations. Recipients of grants have included state government agencies, community coalitions, private health care systems, professional societies, labor unions, employers, and research organizations. A complete listing of grant recipients is provided in Exhibit 6.1.

⎯ Recent Research Advances

Through the efforts of the Workers' Compensation Health Initiative, NIOSH, the Workers' Compensation Research Initiative, several state workers' compensation agencies, and independent researchers, new information is beginning to emerge that provides a better picture of the key factors determining the cost and the quality of workers' compensation medical care. Some findings from the new research are:

Impact of Managed Care

Studies from Florida, New Hampshire, Oregon, Washington, and other states have indicated that the use of managed care techniques in workers' compensation saves money, but that patient satisfaction with care is diminished.[4] The evidence is inconclusive as to whether the use of managed care in workers' compensation affects medical and functional outcomes. Studies suggest that managed care can save as much as 20 to 30 percent, mainly through the introduction of discounted fee schedules, decreased utilization of medical services, and a lower incidence and duration of indemnity claims. For example, investigators in a WCHI-sponsored evaluation of Washington State's managed care pilot program found that the mean medical cost per injury declined 21.5 percent, but that 11 percent fewer patients expressed satisfaction with their care, particularly access to their medical providers.[5] Preliminary results of data from research conducted by the Workers' Compensation Research Institute indicate that restricting care to designated networks of medical providers can decrease medical costs by 15 to 40 percent.[6]

Cost Drivers

Considerable effort has been directed toward gaining a better understanding of what drives the costs of workers' compensation medical care. Several studies have documented that such costs are greater than costs for similar disorders treated under general health care plans.[7] The difference has been attributed to the greater utilization of health care providers and medical services in workers' compensation cases—a utilization that is presumably linked to the need for supplementing traditional care with therapies and treatments that facilitate functional recovery and hasten the employee's return to work. Economists have identified other factors that may account for the cost differential, including the lack of patient cost sharing, the tendency for HMOs under capitated payment plans to shift cases and costs to the more lucrative fee-for service reimbursement normally available for workers' compensation cases, and financial incentives motivating workers to exaggerate their symptoms or extend their disability periods.[8]

Communication

A variety of studies have documented the importance of communication among patients, employers, providers, and workers' compensation insurers throughout the course of treatment for occupational injuries and illnesses, including rehabilitation and the return to work.[9] Breakdowns in communications have been shown to result in delayed treatment, increased litigation, inappropriate care, and unsuccessful return to work. New communications tools and procedures, such as the standardized Uniform Workability Reporting Form, developed by the WCHI-supported Mid-America Coalition on Health Care, in Kansas City, are showing promise in improving communication between parties and eliminating barriers to care. The use of specially trained nurse case managers has been touted as an effective way of improving communication and the coordination of care in workers' compensation.[10] A new investigation of "enhanced" case management protocols for federal employees—involving patient education, improved communication with the employer, and a coordinated effort to redesign jobs to fit the restricted abilities of injured workers—has recently been launched in a WCHI-funded study led by researchers from Georgetown University.

Integration of Workers' Compensation with Other Medical Care and Disability Programs

Pilot programs in California, Maine, Oregon and other states have explored the feasibility of coordinating or integrating medical care and wage replacement benefits available through workers' compensation with other private and public health insurance and disability benefits programs. The effort to establish such state-regulated "24-hour coverage" programs has proved to be technically challenging and politically difficult. Low enrollment in pilot programs impeded WCHI-sponsored research projects in California and Maine. At the same time, market-driven private sector initiatives blending disability and medical care plans for both work-related and nonoccupational conditions continue to evolve. The Minnesota Health Partnership, another WCHI grant recipient, has implemented a project of this type at several primary care clinics in the Minneapolis area. Employers participating in the project have established a coordinated plan in which medical providers evaluate the limitations on patients' work activity and offer disability management guidance, whether the condition is work-related or not. For example, physicians assess the ability of patients with diabetes, arthritis, asthma, and other common conditions to perform vocational activities like lifting, carrying, operating machinery, and working in proximity to industrial chemicals. They then advise employers and employees about limitations on work activities and appropriate job modifications. Research studies to assess the impact of this program on patients' health status and vocational performance are now under way.

Expanded Assessment of Health Care Outcomes

Traditional investigations of workers' compensation medical care have focused relatively narrowly on evaluating direct medical costs and the amount of time needed for return to work. However, several recent studies have demonstrated the inadequacy of relying on these limited conceptions of medical care outcomes in workers' compensation cases.[11] It has been argued that how quickly a patient returns to work is a misleading indicator of health care effectiveness, because the first return to work is often followed by subsequent episodes of work disability; one study estimated it occurred 61 percent of the time.[12] For these reasons, suggestions have been made for new methods to assess not only the direct economic results of work injuries but also their indirect consequences on vocational and social function, quality of life, psychological well-being and satisfaction with care, risk of reinjury, subsequent labor market experiences, and other functional outcomes.[13] NIOSH recently awarded grants for a variety of studies that have examined an assortment of such indirect outcomes.[14] Numerous new research instruments have been developed to measure these outcomes, including adaptations of standardized tools for assessing health status and quality of life; questionnaires on work limitations; devices to evaluate functional capacity; and approaches for evaluating residual pain, impairment, and impact on vocational performance. In the spring of 1999, NIOSH and WCHI cosponsored a national conference on these issues entitled "Functional, Economic, and Social Outcomes of Occupational Injuries and Illnesses: Integrating Social, Economic, and Health Services Research."[15]

Rehabilitation and Return to Work

Significant strides have been made in identifying many of the factors that contribute to a successful recovery and return to work following occupational injuries and illnesses. Some recent studies have suggested that a "sports medicine" approach featuring early intervention and aggressive physical therapy is effective in facilitating a shortened course of disability.[16] Other studies have found that workplace accommodations and transitional duty assignments represent an effective strategy for a successful return to work. Scientists have recently described numerous predictors for the recovery of vocational function, including personal motivation and job satisfaction, social support mechanisms, mental health status, and organizational factors like job stress, supervisory support, work pace, employer size, and employment practices.[17] An increasing number of medical authorities have suggested that early return to work and a prompt resumption of limited physical activity following low back injuries and other musculoskeletal disorders can help maintain functional capacity and minimize long-term impairment.[18] This approach has been incorporated into the new treatment guidelines for the management of work-related musculoskeletal conditions recently released by the American College of Occupational and Environmental Medicine.[19] Similar guidelines have been promulgated by several state workers' compensation agencies. WCHI-funded research studies are being conducted to evaluate clinicians' acceptance and use of these guidelines, and the impact on quality and functional outcomes of the mandatory practice guidelines issued by the Minnesota Department of Labor and Industry.

Underreporting and Other Barriers to Access

Despite the promise of a no-fault system offering comprehensive medical benefits with no patient copayments, many injured workers face significant difficulties in obtaining appropriate and timely care. Recent research has begun to document the extent and nature of the problem. A growing body of evidence suggests that many injured workers may be reluctant to report work-related ailments owing to fear of employer reprisal, concern about losing their jobs, employer safety incentive programs that reward low claims frequency rates, language and cultural barriers, and lack of knowledge about the availability of workers' compensation benefits.[20] In some states, low fee schedules discourage doctors from accepting workers' compensation cases. Several studies have shown that despite the full benefits supposedly available, workers often incur significant out-of-pocket expenses in order to obtain treatment for workplace injuries.[21] Many jurisdictions do not provide coverage for all occupational diseases. The federal Department of Energy, for example, has advocated federal legislation that would provide for treatment of workers suffering from beryllium poisoning contracted at government weapons sites. Preliminary evidence from several states indicates that barriers to workers' compensation care do not affect all workers equally, and that ethnic and racial minorities, the working poor, immigrants and migrant workers, and teenagers are particularly vulnerable to workplace health hazards and inferior access to care.[22]

—— Emerging Trends and Policy Implications

As more information is acquired, concerns have mounted about whether cost containment strategies and recent legislative reforms jeopardize the quality of care provided to injured workers. Mistrust and litigation still pervade the system, and workers, employers, health care providers, and policy makers remain confused and frustrated about how to identify and obtain the best possible care. Several approaches are being considered for continuing to improve workers' compensation medical care.

Accountability

Considerable interest has been expressed in devising ways to hold managed care organizations accountable for providing high-quality care to workers receiving treatment for occupational disorders. Some states, such as California, Florida, and Oregon, have adopted certification requirements for managed care organizations that have established contracts with purchasers (employers or insurers) to provide medical services for injured workers covered under workers' compensation. Industry groups have developed accreditation standards for workers' compensation provider networks and utilization management programs. Model language to ensure the quality of care for use in contracts between purchasers and managed care organizations providing workers' compensation medical care were recently proposed in a study sponsored by the National Association of Insurance Commissioners.[23] The American Accreditation Health Care Commission, in a new project funded by WCHI, is leading an effort to develop a set of performance measurement standards for managed care organizations treating patients covered by workers' compensation, similar to the health care standards developed for health maintenance organizations by the National Committee for Quality Assurance. Most authorities contend that no single strategy for assuring quality-of-care will be sufficient by itself, but that a multifaceted approach drawing on market mechanisms, regulation, and self-regulatory methods will be needed.

Defining the Quality of Care

All such efforts to ensure quality are impeded by the lack of agreement about what constitutes high-quality workers' compensation medical care. Unlike the general health care arena, there are few generally accepted clinical measures by which to quantify the effectiveness of treatment in the most common workers' compensation cases. Employers and workers still argue about the relative importance of cost control and expedited return to work, and medical authorities are split about basic aspects of care, such as the advisability of rest or activity for recovery from low back pain. More research is needed that will broaden the assessment of outcomes beyond cost and return-to-work to include a wide range of health status and functional indicators, indirect social and economic consequences, and medical services utilization.

Inadequacies of Existing Data

Until recently, the paucity of available data limited the research options. Historically, there have not been any standardized data collection protocols or instruments available for use in this field. Most studies have relied on claims administration databases maintained by insurers or state workers' compensation agencies. These were restricted primarily to basic payment and transactional information. Few data sources contained detailed information on utilization of medical services, health status, or workers' experiences with care.

During the past few years, prompted in part by the grant initiatives described above, state agencies and research institutions have launched studies that incorporate worker self-reported survey data, medical records review, and expanded reporting by health care systems. Projects have been initiated to enlarge the use of computerized accident reporting and electronic data interchange, and to compile the resulting information into usable research databases. A large consortium of researchers directed by investigators at the University of Texas-Houston School of Public Health was recently awarded a WCHI grant to conduct a planning and feasibility study aimed at devising a standardized research methodology for use in the creation of a national database for the study of workers' compensation medical care.

Dissemination of Information to Key Individuals and Groups

It is difficult for injured workers, employers, insurers, health care systems, medical providers, and state policy makers to obtain information about workers' compensation medical care. Although some insurers, state agencies, and health care institutions provide information about workers' compensation medical care, there are currently no centralized agencies or clearinghouses (other than the WCHI) focusing on this issue. To address this need, the WCHI awarded two grants in 1999 to establish model resource centers in Rhode Island and California to collect and disseminate information about how to improve workers' compensation medical care. These centers, housed in state workers' compensation agencies, will help form broadly based stakeholder interest groups; acquire and release relevant state-specific data; conduct educational workshops and conferences; and disseminate information through Internet websites and other media. These models could help stimulate the creation of similar resource centers in other states and nationally.

Interaction of Workers' Compensation and Other Health Care Programs

Recent studies suggest that care delivered under workers' compensation is not independent of care provided through other health care systems.[24] For example, the working poor, especially transient and part-time workers, may fluctuate between participation in workers' compensation and Medicaid programs. Individuals suffering chronic disabilities as the result of work injuries may end up receiving disability benefits from Social Security. As many as 11 percent of patients receiving care at community-based free clinics may be there because of work-related conditions.[25] Although many small employers do not offer health plans to their employees, most have to carry workers' compensation insurance, thereby creating a potential incentive for otherwise uninsured employees to frame their medical problems as work-related. These cross-system effects could have significant implications for health care policy and the design of health and disability insurance systems. To date, however, these issues have received limited attention from researchers and government policy makers. They constitute an important area for research that needs increased consideration.

⟿ At the Convergence of Work and Health

Workers' compensation medical care is part of a larger dynamic involving the interplay between workers' employment experiences and their health. The occurrence of occupational injuries and illnesses is a clear indication of how work can affect health. But evidence is accumulating that job conditions and workplace demands may also play a role in coronary heart disease, hypertension, asthma, psychological disorders, and a variety of other common conditions.[26] Likewise, workers' health status and physical impairments can affect their productivity and job experiences.[27] Little is currently known about the complex connections between work, health, and workers' health care.

Further study is needed to investigate working conditions as one of many interrelated social determinants of population health. Because of the inherent linkages among occupational disorders, health care, and the management of work and functional disabilities, the workers' compensation system can shed light more broadly on methods for enhancing chronic care and supportive services for people with restricted functional capacities.

New knowledge about the ways that work affects health (and vice versa) challenges old notions about the supposed rigid distinction between occupational and nonoccupational disorders, upon which the workers' compensation insurance system is based. If employment conditions can influence and help determine a wide variety of common ailments, then an integrated insurance plan and medical care arrangement covering all employee maladies, regardless of cause, might help foster greater continuity of care and decreased fragmentation of prevention, health promotion, and rehabilitation efforts. Likewise, techniques that have been honed in the occupational medicine field for managing workers' disabilities and facilitating job accommodation for persons with physical and functional impairments have great promise for transference into the general health setting and stimulating new employment-based public health initiatives. Experience gained through the Workers' Compensation Health Initiative is helping to open the door into this new area of potentially great significance for employers, policy makers, and all those interested in the promotion of workers' health.

Notes

1. R. Herbert, K. Janeway, and C. Schechter. "Carpal Tunnel Syndrome and Workers' Compensation Among an Occupational Clinic Population in New York State." *American Journal of Industrial Medicine*, 1999, *35*, 335–342.
2. See A. E. Dembe. "Access to Medical Care for Occupational Disorders: Difficulties and Disparities." *Journal of Health and Social Policy*, 2000 (in press).
3. D. Milton, G. Solomon, R. Rosiello, and R. Herrick. "Risk and Incidence of Asthma Attributable to Occupational Exposure Among HMO Members," *American Journal of Industrial Medicine* 1998, *33*, 1–10.
4. A. E. Dembe. "Evaluating the Impact of Managed Health Care in Workers' Compensation." In J. Harris, (ed.), *Managed Care*. Philadelphia: Hanley & Belfus, 1998, pp. 799–821.
5. K. B. Kyes, T. M. Wickizer, G. Franklin, et al. "Evaluation of the Washington State Workers' Compensation Managed Care Pilot Program I: Medical Outcomes and Patient Satisfaction." *Medical Care*, 1999, *37*, 972–981; A. Cheadle, T. M. Wickizer, G. Franklin, et al. "Evaluation of the Washington

State Workers' Compensation Managed Care Pilot Program II: Medical and Disability Costs." *Medical Care*, 1999, *37*, 982–993.

6. W. G. Johnson, M. L. Baldwin, and S. C. Marcus. *The Impact of Workers' Compensation Networks on Medical Costs and Disability Payments.* Cambridge, Mass.: Workers' Compensation Research Institute, 1999.

7. W. G. Johnson, J. F. Burton Jr., L. Thornquist, and B. Zaldman. "Why Does Workers' Compensation Pay More for Health Care?" *Benefits Quarterly*, 1993, Fourth Quarter, 22–31; W. G. Johnson, M. L. Baldwin, and J. F. Burton Jr. "Why is the Treatment of Work-Related Injuries So Costly? New Evidence From California." *Inquiry*, 1996, *33*, 53–65.

8. R. J. Butler, R. P. Hartwig, and H. Gardner. "HMOs, Moral Hazard and Cost Shifting in Workers' Compensation." *Journal of Health Economics*, 1997, *16*, 191–206.

9. Intracorp. *Intracorp Injured Workers Study: The Workers' Compensation Experience.* Philadelphia: Intracorp, July, 1997; J. Sum. *Navigating the California Workers' Compensation System: The Injured Worker's Experience.* San Francisco: California Commission on Health and Safety, 1996.

10. K. J. Martin. "Workers' Compensation: Case Management Strategies." AAOHN Journal, 1995, *43*, 245–250; Response Analysis Corporation. *Middle Market Case Management Study: Report on Using Case Management in Workers' Compensation.* Princeton, N.J.: American International Group Claims Services, 1996.

11. J. S. Himmelstein and G. Pransky. "Measuring and Improving the Quality of Workers' Compensation Medical Care." *Workers' Compensation Monitor*, 1995, *8*, 4–9; M. L. Baldwin, W. G. Johnson, and R. J. Butler. "The Error of Using Returns-to-Work to Measure the Outcomes of Health Care." *American Journal of Industrial Medicine*, 1996, *29*, 632–641; G. Pransky and J. Himmelstein. "Outcomes Research: Implications for Occupational Health." *American Journal of Industrial Medicine*, 1996, *29*, 573–583.

12. M. L. Baldwin, W. G. Johnson, and R. J. Butler. "The Error of Using Returns-to-Work to Measure the Outcomes of Health Care." *American Journal of Industrial Medicine*, 1996, *29*, 632–641.

13. G. Pransky and J. Himmelstein. "Outcomes Research: Implications for Occupational Health." *American Journal of Industrial Medicine*, 1996, *29*, 573–583.

14. G. Pransky, K. Benjamin, C. Hill-Fatouhi, et al. "Outcomes in Work-Related Upper Extremity and Low Back Injuries: Results of a Retrospective Study." *American Journal of Industrial Medicine*, 2000, *37*, 400–409; T. Morse, C. Dillon, N. Warren, et al. "The Economic and Social Consequences of Work-Related Musculoskeletal Disorders: The Connecticut Upper-Extremity

Surveillance Project (CUSP)." *International Journal of Occupational and Environmental Health,* 1998, *4,* 209–216; J. Keogh, I. Nuwayhid, J. Gordon, et al. "The Impact of Occupational Injury on Injured Worker and Family: Outcomes of Upper Extremity Cumulative Trauma Disorders in Maryland Workers." *American Journal of Industrial Medicine,* 2000, (in press).

15. See G. Pransky, K. Benjamin, and A. Dembe. "Performance and Quality Measurement in Occupational Health Services: Current Status and Agenda for Further Research." In the *Proceedings of the NIOSH/RWJF Conference: Functional, Economic, and Social Outcomes of Occupational Injuries and Illnesses: Integrating Social, Economic, and Health Services Research.* Denver, Colorado: NIOSH, June, 1999.

16. T. Parry and W. P. Molmen. *Return to Productivity.* San Francisco: Integrated Benefits Institute, 1996.

17. A. Dembe. *The Social Consequences of Occupational Injuries and Illnesses,* Working paper, Worcester, Mass.: UMass Center for Health Policy and Research, 1999.

18. B. G. Margoshes and B. S. Webster. "Why Do Occupational Injuries Have Different Health Outcomes?" In T. G. Mayer, R. J. Gatchel, and P. B. Polatin (eds.), *Occupational Musculoskeletal Disorders: Function, Outcomes, and Evidence.* Philadelphia: Lippencott, Williams and Wilkins, 2000, pp. 47–61.

19. J. S. Harris. "The ACOEM Occupation Medicine Practice Guidelines." In Harris J. S., Loeppke R. R. (eds.), *Integrated Health Management: The Key role of Occupational Medicine in Managed Care, Disability Management and Integrated Delivery Systems.* Beverly Farms, Mass.: OEM Press, 1998.

20. G. Pransky, T. Snyder, A. Dembe et al. "Under-reporting of Work-related Disorders in the Workplace: A Case Study and Review of the Literature." *Ergonomics,* 1999, *42,* 171–182; J. Biddle, K. Roberts, K. D. Rosenman et al. "What Percentage of Workers with Work-Related Illnesses Receive Workers' Compensation Benefits?" *Journal of Occupational and Environmental Medicine,* 1998, *40,* 325–331.

21. G. Pransky, K. Benjamin, C. Hill-Fatouhi et al. "Outcomes in Work-Related Upper Extremity and Low Back Injuries: Results of a Retrospective Study," *American Journal of Industrial Medicine,* 2000, *37,* 400–409; T. Morse, C. Dillon, N. Warren, et al. "The Economic and Social Consequences of Work-Related Musculoskeletal Disorders: The Connecticut Upper-Extremity Surveillance Project (CUSP)." *International Journal of Occupational and Environmental Health,* 1998, *4,* 209–216.

22. A. E. Dembe, "Access to Medical Care for Occupational Disorders: Difficulties and Disparities." *Journal of Health and Social Policy,* 2000, (in press).

23. A. E. Dembe and J. S. Himmelstein. "Contract Provisions to Ensure Quality in Workers' Compensation Managed Care Arrangements." *Journal of Insurance Regulation*, 1999, *18*, 289–326.

24. M. J. Graetz and J. L. Mashaw. *True Security: Rethinking American Social Insurance.* New Haven: Yale University Press, 1999; D. Mont, J. F. Burton, and V. Reno. *Workers' Compensation: Benefits, Coverage, and Costs, 1997–1998, New Estimates.* Washington, D.C.: National Academy of Social Insurance, 2000.

25. A. E. Dembe, J. Johnstone, and A. J. Ramler. "Improving Access to Workers' Compensation Health Care for Underserved Populations in Worcester, Massachusetts." Working paper, Worcester, Mass.: UMass Center for Health Policy and Research, 1999.

26. S. A. Stansfeld, R. Fuhrer, J. Head, J. Ferrie, and M. Shipley. "Work and Psychiatric Disorder in the Whitehall II Study." *Journal of Psychosomatic Research*, 1997, *43*, 73–81; R. Peter and J. Siegrist. "Chronic Work Stress, Sickness Absence, and Hypertension in Middle Managers: General or Specific Sociological Explanations." *Social Science and Medicine*, 1997, *45*, 1111–1120; M. G. Marmot, H. Bosma, J. Hemingway, E. Brunner, and S. Stansfeld. "Contribution of Job Control and Other Risk Factors to Social Variations in Coronary Heart Disease Incidence." *Lancet*, 1997, *350*, 235–239.

27. W. N. Burton, D. J. Conti, C. Chen, A. B Schultz, and D. W Edington. "The Role of Health Risk Factors and Disease on Worker Productivity." *Journal of Occupational and Environmental Medicine*, 1999, *40*, 863–877; I. M. Cockburn, H. L. Bailit, E. R. Berndt, and S. N. Finkelstein. "Loss of Work Productivity Due to Illness and Medical Treatment." *Journal of Occupational and Environmental Medicine*, 1999, *41*, 948–953.

Exhibit 6.1. Workers' Compensation Health Initiative.

First Round Grantees

Lead Agency: State of Maine Bureau of Insurance
Project Name: Twenty-Four-Hour Coverage Pilot Project
Grant Amount: $250,000

This project involved the development of a 24-hour coverage pilot project in Maine, based on enabling legislation enacted in 1995.

Lead Agency: New York State Department of Civil Service
Project Name: OneCard Rx
Grant Amount: $253,282

The New York State Department of Civil Service developed and implemented an integrated workers' compensation and health insurance prescription drug program for New York State employees.

Lead Agency: Institute for Research and Education, HealthSystem Minnesota
Project Name: Minnesota Health Partnership: Coordinated Health Care and Disability Management
Grant Amount: $254,270

The Minnesota Health Partnership, a diverse community coalition, created a coordinated health care delivery model which blends traditional employee health care and workers' compensation medical coverage, along with disability management protocols for all patients.

Lead Agency: Mid-America Coalition on Health Care
Project Name: Cooperative Employer-Provider Medical Management & Early Return to Work
Grant Amount: $270,439

This community-based coalition in Kansas City, Missouri, developed new communications tools for improving care, including a standardized workability reporting form, along with employer and provider protocols for care.

Lead Agency: American College of Occupational and Environmental Medicine
Project Name: Occupational Medicine Practice Guidelines for Medical & Disability Management
Grant Amount: $121,560

This grant supported the initial dissemination and adoption of the occupational practice guidelines recently developed by the American College of Occupational and Environmental Medicine.

Exhibit 6.1.   Workers' Compensation Health Initiative, *continued.*

First Round Grantees

Lead Agency:	Union of Needletrades, Industrial and Textile Employees (UNITE)
Project Name:	UNITE Occupational Health/Workers' Compensation Program
Grant Amount:	$263,138

UNITE devised new methods for ensuring union members had access to medical care for work-related disorders without regard to claims denial by insurance carriers or legal adjudication of the claim.

Lead Agency:	The Electrical Employers Self-Insurance Safety Plan (EESISP)
Project Name:	The Comprehensive and Organized Managed Care Program (COMP)
Grant Amount:	$374,094

This project involved the development of a negotiated union-management health plan that provides 24-hour health care and coordinated disability benefits for electrical workers in the New York City area.

Lead Agency:	UCLA Center for Health Policy Research
Project Name:	Evaluation of California's 24-Hour Pilot Program
Grant Amount:	$458,994

Research was conducted to evaluate California's 24-hour coverage pilot programs adopted under 1993 authorizing legislation.

Lead Agency:	University of Washington
Project Name:	Washington State Workers' Compensation Managed Care Pilot Evaluation
Grant Amount:	$252,768

This research study evaluated the Washington State Managed Care Pilot Project which featured experience rated, capitated premiums and occupational medicine networks for workers' compensation.

Lead Agency:	Stratus Health
Project Name:	Minnesota Mandatory Treatment Parameters Evaluation
Grant Amount:	$386,709

The study examined provider compliance with Minnesota's treatment parameters and their effect on costs, quality of care, functional and social outcomes, satisfaction, and return to work.

♪♪

Exhibit 6.1.   Workers' Compensation Health Initiative, *continued.*

Second Round Grantees

Lead Agency:	American Accreditation Health Care Commission
Project Name:	Development of a Performance Measurement Set for Workers' Compensation Managed Care Organizations
Grant Amount:	$393,638

This project involves the development and pilot testing of a set of standard performance measures for workers' compensation managed care organizations.

Lead Agency:	Champlain Valley Physicians Hospital Medical Center
Project Name:	North Country On the Job Network: A Rural Coalition Accessing Medical Management for Injured Workers
Grant Amount:	$319,559

Through a community-based coalition, a unique health care delivery model for management of injured workers in a rural region of upstate New York is being implemented and evaluated.

Lead Agency:	Georgetown University Medical Center
Project Name:	Enhanced Case Management for Workers Covered Under the Federal Employees Compensation Act
Grant Amount:	$481,104

This project involves the development and testing of a multifaceted case management model that enhances the approach currently used in the federal workers' compensation system.

Lead Agency:	Institute for Research and Education, HealthSystem Minnesota
Project Name:	Evaluation of the Minnesota Health Partnership: Coordinated Health Care and Disability Management
Grant Amount:	$499,986

This research study is evaluating the effectiveness of the Minnesota Health Partnership, an ongoing project aimed at establishing coordinated medical delivery and disability management.

Lead Agency:	Maine Medical Assessment Foundation
Project Name:	Maine Workers' Compensation Health Care Improvement Initiative
Grant Amount:	$205,440

This project involves the formation of a stakeholder study group, the design and development of a centralized state workers' compensation health care database, and the implementation and testing of a program for routine functional assessment in the workplace.

Exhibit 6.1.   Workers' Compensation Health Initiative, *continued.*

Second Round Grantees

Lead Agency: New School for Social Research

Project Name: Evaluating the Benefits of Enhanced Access to Medical
                     Care for Patients at UNITE's Union Health Center.

Grant Amount: $217,752

This research project is evaluating the health care delivery and financing
innovations recently established at New York City's Union Health Center
by UNITE.

Lead Agency: New York Department of Civil Service

Project Name: Evaluation of OneCard Rx Integrated Prescription Drug
                     Program

Grant Amount: $334,323

This evaluation study is examining the impact of the recently initiated
OneCard Rx program, which allows New York State employees to use a single
prescription drug benefit plan for both workers' compensation and general
(nonoccupational) health care.

Lead Agency: University of Colorado Health Sciences Center

Project Name: Evaluation of the Acceptance and Use of ACOEM
                     ACOEM Treatment Guidelines

Grant Amount: $221,719

This multistate, multiclinic study by researchers from the University of Colorado Health Sciences Center is exploring clinicians' acceptance and use of
the recently released American College of Occupational and Environmental
Medicine practice guidelines.

Third Round Grantees

Lead Agency: State of Rhode Island Department of Labor and Training

Project Name: Development of a Model State Technical Resource Center
                     for the Improvement of Workers' Compensation Medical
                     Care

Grant Amount: $267,500

The state of Rhode Island, with input from key stakeholder groups, will
establish a model state technical resource center for the improvement of
workers' compensation medical care.

c/f&

Exhibit 6.1. Workers' Compensation Health Initiative, *continued.*

Third Round Grantees

Lead Agency: California Public Health Institute

Project Name: Planning and Development of the California Work
                  Injury Resource Center

Grant Amount: $81,079

This one-year planning grant will support initial planning activities for the
establishment of the California Work Injury Resource Center for the
improvement of workers' compensation medical care.

Lead Agency: The University of Texas—Houston School of Public
                  Health

Project Name: Development and Testing of a Standardized Method for
                  Creating an Interstate Database for the Study of Workers'
                  Compensation Medical Care

Grant Amount: $350,265

The project involves a preliminary planning and feasibility study for establishing a uniform data-collection methodology that can be applied in creating a national research database for studying outcomes and the quality of
workers' compensation medical care.

CHAPTER SEVEN

—⁓— Sound Partners for Community Health

Digby Diehl

Editors' Introduction

Over the past several years, the Internet has captured the attention of Americans. Health-related websites, capable of providing a wealth of health care information for the "connected" population, seem to spring up on a weekly basis. The potential of the Internet should not, however, obscure the contribution made by a more traditional means of communications that continues to reach millions of Americans—local radio.

To help local radio stations improve their health care programming and have more impact in their listening areas, The Robert Wood Johnson Foundation teamed up with the Benton Foundation to develop, in 1996, a national program called Sound Partners for Community Health. In an unusual twist, a local radio station, to be eligible for funding, needed to collaborate with a community organization, working in a field such as children's health, welfare reform, or end-of-life care.

In this chapter, Digby Diehl, a free-lance journalist and previous contributor to The Robert Wood Johnson Foundation *Anthology*, tells the story of the Sound Partners program, largely as seen through the eyes of some of the 59 grantees and their partners. Unlike many Robert Wood Johnson Foundation-funded programs, which attempt to affect policy at national or state levels and which take place in large metropolitan areas, most of the activity of Sound Partners occurs in small towns and rural areas of America. The story that Diehl recounts is one of *local* public radio and *local* institutions, and the way in which they combine their forces to raise awareness of health issues and bring about change in their own communities.

Over the three years that the program has been in existence, some Sound Partners' grantees have won awards. These include two from the National Federation of Community Broadcasters: KDNA of Granger, Washington, won the Community Impact Award for "Access to Health Care in Yakima Valley" and KGNU of Boulder, Colorado, won the Golden Reel Award for Best Local and Public Affairs Program for "Seeking a Good Death." Other winners include WBST in Muncie, Indiana, which won the Edward R. Murrow Regional Award for Overall News Excellence from the Radio & Television News Directors Association for its series "Living with Death," and KSTX of San Antonio, Texas, which won the Media Award from the Texas Public Health Association for its series "Caring for the Children of Children: Teen Pregnancy in San Antonio."

This chapter complements three other chapters on communications that have appeared in The Robert Wood Johnson Foundation *Anthology*: Frank Karel's retrospective look at the Foundation's global communications strategies elsewhere in this volume, Victoria Weisfeld's examination of the Foundation's radio and television grants in the 1998-1999 *Anthology*, and Marc Kaplan and Mark Goldberg's analysis of how research on managed care was presented to the media in the 1997 *Anthology*.

✌

---

*When I wake up in the morning, it's the first thing I think about—
how am I going to get to it? I have to be alone . . . I have to strategically plan it out . . . just enough time, right? Then there has to be
a secluded bathroom, away from everything, so no one will walk in
on me. It's sick, but it gets my adrenaline pumping. Somehow it ful-
fills me, but it's an addiction like so many others have. You don't
realize how steep a hill it is that you're gonna have to climb back up
to get out of the hell that you've created for yourself. It's a place that's
untouched. It's . . . It's so dark and so lonely that no one . . . no one
is allowed there. It could be the happiest moment in my life and yet
I'm thinking, how can I get my hands on that food, and then, how
can I get it out of me without anyone noticing?*

    *How can I lower myself to this disease that I look at as a disease
for losers? I give in to that voice that tells me I'm a failure. I run to
that addiction that allows me to escape from myself. That's what
I'm really afraid of—facing myself. I'm failing myself by doing this.
Love is an emotion that's so hard for me to feel, because I can't feel
it for myself, so I'll give in to my addiction because it makes me
feel* strong.

—Teenage girl battling bulimia, reading from her diary
What You Don't Know: Youth Speaks Out
KZYX&Z, Mendocino County, California

T his excerpt was generated on a radio show sponsored
by Sound Partners for Community Health, a national program for
public radio stations paired with local community health organizations. Administered by the Benton Foundation and funded by The
Robert Wood Johnson Foundation, the program has two major goals:

- To increase public awareness of specific health issues; and
- To facilitate citizen involvement in making decisions that affect
  health care.

Mainstream resources, such as traditional health care providers, TV, newspapers, and the Internet, are directed at the broad American population; public radio, however, is able to tailor its programming to reach smaller numbers of specific individuals and groups. The Sound Partners program uses the power of radio to aim health and wellness programming at groups who may not have good access to health care or health care information. Most are isolated in one fashion or another from mainstream health information providers. This isolation may have physical, psychological, and/or socioeconomic components—illiteracy, social custom, age, language barrier, fear, poverty, legal status, and geography can all serve to separate people from what they need to know. Community health organizations, the other half of the Sound Partners partnership, participate both in the preparation of broadcast materials and in reaching out to listeners to follow up on the issues covered on the air.

The Robert Wood Johnson Foundation's participation in the Sound Partners program grew out of its long involvement with National Public Radio.[1] In 1994, it supported a program through NPR called "Critical Decision," which assisted local stations in their efforts to cover the issue of health care reform and to conduct outreach activities. The Sound Partners program was intended to go beyond this single topic. Designed to improve the coverage of health care issues where it was weakest—at the local level—Sound Partners attempts to identify important health care issues in communities; inform and stimulate public dialogue; build capacity to conduct effective outreach; and build partnerships between radio stations and local health care organizations.

Overseeing the Sound Partners program for the Benton Foundation is Anne Green, Director of Grantmaking Programs. "The Benton Foundation believes that communications is the driver of social change," she says. "We're trying to use the media to activate citizens, to get them involved with issues." Jointly heading the Sound Partners program at the national level are Mark Sachs, president of Mark Sachs & Associates, a management consulting firm, and Beth Mastin, president of MasComm, a communications consulting firm.

The Sound Partners program—a $2 million five-year initiative—rolled out in two rounds. The Call for Proposals for round 1 was sent, in 1997, to the 400-plus public radio stations supported by the Corporation for Public Broadcasting, or CPB, and the first grants were awarded in October of that year. From more than 100 applicants, 35 recipients were selected; grants ranged from $15,000 to $35,000. A Call for Proposals was issued for the second round, and thirty-three round 2 grantees were notified in January, 2000, of awards for programming that run from August 2000 to August 2001.

In the first round, Sound Partners targeted four general health issues that could be explored by grant recipients. Stations and their partners were free to apply for funding in any area they preferred:

- Children's health
- Youth substance abuse
- End-of-life decisions, and
- Health care and welfare reform

Of the 35 grantees in round 1, nine dealt with children's health, nine with youth substance abuse, seven with end-of-life decisions, and ten with health care and welfare reform.

In the Call for Proposals for the second round, another issue— aging and chronic disease—was added. In addition, the category of health care and welfare reform was changed to the health care safety net. Of the 32 grantees in round 2, six are dealing with children's health, ten with youth substance abuse, five with end-of-life decisions, seven with the health care safety net, and five with aging and chronic disease. By design, the number of returning grantees was limited in order to give additional stations an opportunity to participate. Thus, 23 of the second-round stations receiving grants are participating in the program for the first time.

The stations involved in Sound Partners reach a varied geographical and cultural cross-section of the United States. Grantees include stations serving Latino farming communities in Washington and California, Native Americans in Alaska, Wisconsin, and Arizona, hardscrabble Appalachian areas in West Virginia and Kentucky, and the diverse ethnic urban populations of New York, Detroit, and Minneapolis.

—— Organizing the Program

The Sound Partners program offers participants great leeway in how they deal with their subject matter and how they work with one another. Various grantees forge their own relationships with partner organizations. "For many years, I did a weekly show called the Activist Report," says Joan Buffington, news director of KVMR in Nevada City, California. "I'm a longtime political activist and longtime health care professional. When I wrote the proposal for the Sound Partners grant, I realized that this was an opportunity to put together my years of experience in both fields. For partners, I selected both the Nevada County Department of Human Services and an organization called FREED, which is a really vital, local non-profit group that serves seniors and the disabled. Working with the county was a tactical choice; it was my hunch from my community organizing experience that this would be advantageous, because they would have good connections. I also knew it could be rather limiting in terms of not being able to do things quickly. I chose FREED because I wanted to balance the county agency with a nonprofit organization that had a good reputation for advocacy."

"I picked the death and dying issue because it was of personal interest to me," says Sam Fuqua of KGNU in Boulder, Colorado. "I immediately started thinking of potential partners. Hospice of Boulder County was known to us, at least informally; we had interviewed people from their organization, and done public service announcements for them. Knowing that it was a well-run, stable organization with a really good reputation in the community made choosing both a partner and an issue easier." "Sam and I had great chemistry because he got it about dying, and from the get-go we had the same philosophy," says Fuqua's partner, Kim Mooney of Hospice of Boulder County. "We had the nerve in the same place, and he was willing to do the same kinds of things we were willing to do. We had the same values."

Technical assistance has been a major component of the work of the national Sound Partners staff, headed by its program directors, Mark Sachs and Beth Mastin. This includes advice and assistance with audio production and story development, as well as training and education for radio staff in the coverage of health topics. Information on how to develop and maintain a website has also been made available. "We provide any kind of technical assistance they ask for," Mastin says. "We encourage the stations and partners to call on us as consultants if and when they run into problems, but we don't meddle. We provide them with a framework and encourage them to do the best job with whatever their vision is. The recipients have produced this huge diversity of wonderful programming and connections to the community—which is what we intended them to do."

National conferences of grantees were held both at the beginning and at the end of the first round—a pattern to be repeated in round 2. At the initial gathering, participants received detailed handbooks, lists of contacts, outreach models, and sample promotional materials, as well as access to a website (www.soundpartners.org) with links to other information providers. Grantees were also encouraged to network with one another as the program proceeded.

Perhaps most valuable, however, the meeting served to solidify the working relationship between the two partners, and to focus them on the program. "The initial conference was very good," says Kim Mooney of Hospice of Boulder County. "The Sound Partners staff brought up a lot of things that they thought we should know, but much of it was more familiar to one partner than another. There were issues discussed that I didn't understand that my partner, Sam Fuqua of KGNU, got right away, and vice versa. Between the two of us we understood what the major pieces were."

The initial gathering also offered participants a chance to fine-tune their programs. "After the kickoff conference, we downscaled some," says Jill Hannum of KZYX&Z of Mendocino County, California, "and even then we didn't downscale enough." Hannum worked with the Mendocino County Youth Project to develop programming on the subject of youth substance abuse. "We were too ambitious. We completely gave up the idea of doing the program twice a month, which had been our original goal."

—— Programming: From Call-Ins to Kids

Sound Partners stations used many different programming formats for their broadcasts. They produced news features that varied in length from one minute to one hour. There were mini-dramas, panel discussions, public service announcements, live broadcasts of town meetings, and call-in programs. They used both experts and members of the community as hosts. Some formats seemed better suited to particular issues. Call-ins, for example, were effective for the children's health and end-of-life issues, because listeners with specific needs could connect with professionals to get direct advice or referrals to agencies that could help.

I am a Mexican woman, and we belong to a culture that has much to be proud of, but we also have a lot to learn. I was married three times, and each time it was a nightmare, but every time one ended, I had feelings of guilt. I grew up in a very ugly family, with an irresponsible father who was an alcoholic, and a wife-beater. I knew at a very young age that I did not want to be like my mother—a maid, prostitute, and punching bag for her husband. I think that it's time that instead of letting our daughters play house and buying them dolls, instead of showing them how to cook for their husbands and being their doormats, it's time that we began to educate them. A woman can be happy without a man, without anyone lending her his name.

Carolina, Hispanic parent
La Placita Bilingüe,
KHDC, Salinas, California

Wading into delicate subjects such as this is a hallmark of Sound Partners programming. "We were not afraid of topics," says Graciela Orozco of KHDC, Salinas, California, which dealt with Children's Health. Orozco hosted a Spanish-language program called *La Placita Bilingüe* [the Bilingual Town Square], which offered a forum for Hispanic families to talk about a wide variety of child-centered issues. In Latin culture, the plaza, or town square, is the traditional place for meeting and exchanging information. "We brought together parents and professionals on the air. We talked about teen sex, about AIDS, about child abuse, about raising children in single-parent households. One of our most popular programs was about circumcision," she says. "Sex is usually taboo as a topic of conversation," Orozco says. "You just don't talk about it, but we had a doctor on the show, and he used all the proper names for anatomical parts. People were comfortable discussing it—we had call after call."

For KGNU in Boulder, Colorado, it wasn't just one program but the entire series on end-of-life decisions that had the potential to make people uncomfortable. KGNU partnered with Hospice of Boulder

County to produce a series on death and dying called *Seeking a Good Death.* "Fear of death is an incredibly intelligent thing, because it will motivate you to wake up and look people in the eye and say you love them," says Kim Mooney of Hospice of Boulder County. "But terror of death, which is what we face today, only makes you avoid the subject. It's like a moat—there is so much terror around death that people don't want to deal with the issue. We have trouble working with the senior centers in Boulder; they're offering weightlifting classes rather than getting-ready-for-dying classes, because our seniors are so groovy."

"We had one fully produced documentary that was very moving, and we had live call-in for the first and last shows," says Sam Fuqua of KGNU. "The middle shows were *Nightline* style, with a short feature to set it up and a panel for the next 25 minutes. The advantage of working with Hospice was that they really knew all the people in the death and dying field. They had great guests."

The Taharah, *a physical and ritual cleansing, is carried out as soon after death as possible. We pour bucket after bucket after bucket of water over various body parts, always with prayers, mostly from* Song of Songs. *After the pouring of the water, we dress the person in a plain white shroud, lift her and carry her into her plain pine box and cover her. With final prayers, we seal up the box and she is ready to be taken into the ground.*

Working with death and dying brings us face-to-face with our own mortality. That's the central reason why many of us have joined the Chevra Kaddisha. *Helping someone die, purifying her, and putting her in her coffin is a profound reminder that this could be me at any time.*

Woman member of the *Chevra Kaddisha,*
the burial society of the Jewish Renewal community,
describing a *Taharah* in progress at a mortuary
Seeking a Good Death
KGNU, Boulder, Colorado

"What the Hospice has been trying to do is gently open the door to the subject in a non-threatening way," Kim Mooney says. "That's where the KGNU series really tried to go. The advantage to us of doing it over the radio was anonymity. People sitting at home alone listening to these stories about dying are going to take them differently from the way they would if they were sitting in a group and had to worry about whether they were crying or not. They don't have to dialogue with you; there's nobody standing there who they think is going to make them engage in conversation. Going into people's homes through the radio in little bits was great. We introduced the topic from a couple of different angles, then talked about how to start thinking about death: What do you do to get ready for it? What are the mechanics of it? What does it mean to pay for it? What kind of care do you get? People got a chance to listen passively without having to worry about having to respond. We were planting seeds."

Stations dealing with similar issues developed a wide variety of approaches to covering the topic. WRTU in Puerto Rico offered thirteen one-hour programs on youth substance abuse. The series was anchored by a quartet of young adolescents, who also were involved in production. "The children brought a lot to these shows," says Luis Luna of WRTU. "They co-hosted with adults, did interviews, and selected music." The station's partner was the Center for Rehabilitation through the Arts. "Using the arts is attractive to children," the center's Jacqueline O'Neill says. "They are not intimidated by art." The two partners capped the series, called *Como Gente Grande* [Like Big People], with Punto de Encuentro, a day-long street fair in San Juan. "In addition to music, dance, and theatre, the carnival had booths, displays of confiscated drug paraphernalia, and demonstrations by the police canine unit," Luna says. "There were also mini workshops, where we involved parents in acquiring skills needed to cope with an environment where drugs are common, and promoted techniques kids need to resist drug offerings."

WRTU staff members had already spelled out the content of each of the station's thirteen shows when they submitted their proposal. For the on-air hosts, they selected younger teens and pre-teens who were the age of those most at risk. In contrast, KZYX&Z in Mendocino worked with older teenagers, primarily high school juniors and seniors who were part of peer counseling programs at local high schools. Partnering with the Mendocino County Youth Project, they produced a series called *What You Don't Know: Youth Speaks Out.* "We really let this be a youth-driven program," says Jill Hannum of KZYX&Z. "And we let them choose the topics. We didn't tell them what to focus on. We asked, 'What touches you? What's hot in your life?' and that's where we certainly got our strongest stuff." The Mendocino peer counselors went way beyond "Just Say No," often putting an unexpected spin on how they chose to deal with substance abuse, and even how they defined it. To them, the addictive behavior of bulimia fit within the rubric of substance abuse, the substance being food.

WBAI's Diana Mason, whose New York City station also worked with adolescents to cover the issue of youth substance abuse, had the same experience. "I learned to trust the kids and let 'em roll," she says. "They took us into places I wouldn't have gone—literally and figuratively." One program explored drug use associated with the very edgy dance club rave scene. "I thought I could come in and tell them how to put a radio show together, but I learned right away that this was not about adults telling kids what to do. It was about us listening to them, sharing skills with them, and supporting them so they could tell their stories on the radio."

WBAI partnered with Global Kids, a group that focuses on developing youth skills in leadership and teamwork. Global Kids "prepares young people as global citizens," says Mason, who decided to partner with the organization after several members appeared on her program, *Healthstyles*. "The kids examined the influence of advertising and the media on teen smoking, and incorporated global perspectives on the marketing of tobacco into the segment. Another show investigated the link between religion and drugs—they looked at Rastafarians and ganja, and at the spiritual uses of wine in the Catholic Church."

"It takes a leap of faith to let young people have a voice," says Jill Hannum's partner, Leslie Rich of the Mendocino County Youth Project. Hannum of KZYX&Z was willing to make that leap, in part because she was prepared. "We had training programs. We had mock shows before they went on, and mock call-ins. By and large, I'd say that 80 percent of the kids acquitted themselves like experts. Most of the problems involved teenage boys. As we know, they mature more slowly and their tongues cleave to the roofs of their mouths for many more years. When there were problems, it was usually that the young men froze on the air, or just didn't have the verbal skills to track the question into an answer. We found that as the program progressed the kids who did the program repeatedly were all young women."

"One of the best programs we did involved a girl who dealt with the subject of methamphetamine in her town," Hannum continues. "It amazed me how much was in the schools, how much influence it had on people's lives, how easy she and the kids she interviewed said it was to get—and how completely the police turned their backs to the situation. The kids didn't know whether the cops were just indifferent to it or whether they couldn't figure out how to deal with meth and eleven-year-olds. She said, 'It's not in the high schools anymore so much; it's in junior high.' Here was this sixteen-year-old saying, 'My group's O.K., but I'm worried about the young people.' She had a lot of anxiety about how her friends would react to her program, but when I spoke with her afterward, she was relieved. She said, 'I thought that I would be ostracized for doing this, but all my fears were for nothing. I thought they would single me out for ratting on them, but people who heard it told me that it reflected the truth.'"

"We are in what they call the emerald triangle—a three-county area where there is a lot of marijuana grown," Leslie Rich says. "Marijuana is part of the subculture here, and the kids grew up in it. For grownups, marijuana cultivation is a viable option as a life choice. Mendocino County is economically depressed, and many kids here have family and friends—basically good people—who grow dope on the side."

"I've had my socks knocked off by the intelligence, the skills, the self-possession and the self-knowledge that most of the young people who have been on the program have displayed," Hannum says. "I've been nothing but impressed. The kids are all right. My only surprise was in the incredible openness that they were willing to display about topics one is told that teens keep their mouths shut about."

—⁓— Preliminary Observations on the Potential of Community Radio Partnerships

1. *Community Radio Partnerships Can Empower People*

KHDC's *La Placita Bilingüe* proved to be empowering for Latino parents. "Parents initially felt that what they had to say was not important," says *La Placita* anchor, Graciela Orozco. "They were intimidated, even parents who were very articulate when I spoke with them one-on-one. Getting them to come on the show required painstaking planning. I had to find them, convince them, talk to them about the topic, and give them an idea what direction the discussion would take. But more than anything, they had to trust me that they're going to be O.K. when they came on the show. The interview had to be constructed so that they were comfortable, so that they knew I wasn't going to put them on the spot. Then there were other things that we had to take care of that we didn't initially foresee, like babysitting and transportation.

"Those kinds of obstacles needed time and money and somebody to stay on top of them, but there was a huge payoff. These parents discovered that they have something to offer, a voice of wisdom about parenting. One of the best examples is Cristina, a young mom in her early 30s. When I first met her, she was part of the parent committee at her school and she would attend meetings, but that was the extent of it. After she signed up to be on the show, I contacted her to confirm, but she didn't have a ride, so I offered to pick her up. Over the period of a year, she became a spokesperson for the Head Start committee and a parent organizer at her school—she's just really blossomed. When you talk about the kind of effect the show had, I see that as a great impact."

The series *Who Cares?* produced by KVMR in Nevada City, California, covered the issue of access to health care. "We're an old Gold Rush town, a tourist area with gorgeous trees and rivers—the kind of place everybody wants to live," says Joan Buffington, who organized the program. "We're dealing with the gentrification issue, with skyrocketing costs of living and no increase in incomes, particularly in the service sector. We have twice the statewide ratio of older people. The Sound Partners program gave KVMR an opportunity to look at who gets health care and the politics of health care. We really focused on the access issue. We empowered listeners by putting them on the air and having providers respond to them."

It wasn't just the listeners who were empowered. The Sound Partners program brought important changes to KVMR, and to Buffington herself. "I'd never written a grant proposal before," she says. "KVMR had received several technical support grants from CPB, but had never been awarded a content-driven grant. It was a real leap forward for the station in terms of supporting the idea of public affairs programming. KVMR had started out as a kind of hippie station. It played a lot of music, but the news and public affairs coverage had been pretty haphazard until the past few years. Some of us who are serious about it have been working to try to do more serious professional work, and in public affairs, it takes a lot of time and effort. The grant enabled me to become news director here. Doing that in addition to doing *Who Cares?* was an overload, but it was a welcome one, because it meant that the station was acknowledging the importance of news and public affairs, and giving the staff time to do that.

"*Who Cares?* accomplished exactly what we wanted it to do, both for KVMR and for the community," Buffington says. "It increased the legitimacy of KVMR as a viable media resource by leaps and bounds. We made many contacts and had an impact on recipients. At least as important, however, was the fact that we made a lot of contacts at the provider level—doctors at the hospital, people in the nonprofits, people in the county government sector, supervisors—people who had never heard of KVMR before. After the year of *Who Cares?* KVMR became recognized, which gave us a legitimacy that has continued. We now have developed a news department and put out some real professional news coverage, so people keep calling with information, and that's real exciting."

2. *Community Radio Partnerships Can Help People Navigate the Health Care System*

"The fact that people had a place they could call in and tell their personal stories was a huge piece of education for everybody," says Kim Mooney of Hospice of Boulder County. "That's how people learn about death and dying—by listening to other people's stories. Anecdotes from other people's lives are 100 percent more effective than a textbook. People are always looking for a place to empathize, and to be able to say, "That happened to me." For most Sound Partners stations, outreach efforts were directed at listeners who needed help with substance abuse, end-of-life, children's health, or health care safety net issues.

KDNA in Granger, Washington, already had a positive relationship with its partner, the Yakima Valley Farm Workers Clinic—a relationship that deepened as they began exploring how to deal with their issue, the health care safety net. They shared not only the same values but a matching constituency—migrant farm workers.

The name Yakima Valley Farm Workers Clinic is perhaps deceptive. Offering services worthy of a small hospital, including routine medical and dental care, mental health and nutritional services, and specialized care such as obstetrics, pediatrics, and internal medicine, this comprehensive clinic employs more than 900 people. "Among the Hispanic population, the incidence of tuberculosis and diabetes is very high," says Ann Gallegos-Northrup, director of operations for the clinic. "For numerous reasons, we have folks who may not necessarily be aware of the implications of their condition. They don't seek care, or they don't follow their doctor's instructions." Just ten minutes away from KDNA, the clinic furnished the station with tapes on numerous important health topics, which were broadcast on a regular schedule. The station also sent reporters to interview health care professionals on topics such as how women's health and the importance of dealing safely with agricultural pesticides. In addition, they reinforced the message that people who were ill had nothing to fear from *la migra*—the federal Immigration and Naturalization Service—in coming forward for medical treatment. Beginning in round 2, the clinic and KDNA will bring health care providers to the station, where they will respond to call-in questions.

3. *Community Radio Partnerships Can Provide Health Services*

Both the radio station KDNA in Granger, Washington, and the Yakima Valley Farm Workers Clinic had been community resources for many years, and both had earned the trust of the largely Latino population of the area. Many farm workers are not literate in either English or Spanish, and a substantial number are not legally in this country. KDNA had long helped residents with programs dealing with English as a second language, as well as citizenship and legal status. Although the state of Washington offers health and welfare services to indigent residents without requiring a green card, undocumented workers were understandably reluctant to apply for benefits, for fear that their information would be handed over to *la migra*. Even those who had taken steps toward legalization were reticent to file for benefits to which they were entitled, for fear of derailing the process.

To allay immigrant fears of deportation, the station and the clinic put together a series of information capsules to educate people about the availability of prenatal care, preventive health screening, the state's Basic Health Plan, and who could legitimately gain access to these services. Moreover, the station involved the state's Department of Social and Health Services, bringing the DSHS on as an additional partner in the program.

"I initiated contact with the head of DSHS," says Ricardo Garcia of KDNA. "We arranged a meeting here in our building with department administrators and local Latino leaders. As a result, the station became a food stamp application processing center. Spanish-speaking representatives of DSHS come here each week to help our residents complete eligibility forms."

"This radio station has basically turned into the community service provider of everything," Beth Mastin says in appreciation. "They offer all kinds of immigrant services. As a result of their programming on health care needs and welfare reform, workers can get the care and benefits they're entitled to."

State of Washington DSHS workers are also posted regularly to the Yakima Valley Farm Workers Clinic, assisting patients in completing health care applications. "It's very helpful to have state workers out-stationed here at our clinic," says Ann Gallegos-Northrup. "When they're here, they can look up a person's eligibility and tell the patient whether they can get benefits or not—on the day of their visit. There is also an individual stationed at our clinic one day a week who explains the new debit cards. The state is doing away with actual food stamps—the paper product—and people from DSHS are here offering education about what the card means and how to use it."

"The Sound Partners program brought our two organizations closer together," Ricardo Garcia says. "We've become plugged into a bigger network of service providers for immigrants and undocumented workers. Our knowledge is continuing to grow. Even if there is no more funding after this cycle, the clinic and the station will continue to work together."

4. Community Radio Partnerships Can Focus Attention on Local Health Issues

At WVPN in Charleston, West Virginia, the outreach coordinator, Mary Pettey, and a producer/reporter, Susan Leffler, started with a savvy awareness of who their listenership really was, and tailored their program, *Health Care at the Crossroads,* accordingly. The primary focal point was a controversial section of West Virginia's newly revised welfare eligibility criteria. When the new regulations went into effect, the state began to count federal Supplemental Security Income (SSI) benefits as income. As a result, thousands of families were purged from the welfare rolls because one member of the household (often a child) was receiving an SSI stipend because of a mental or physical disability, thus making the family "too rich" to collect welfare benefits.

"We understood that people who were going to be directly affected by the cuts in welfare benefits would not be the people who were listening to public radio in our state," Pettey says. "We aired pieces and did call-in programs knowing, on the other hand, that legislators and policy makers *do* listen to public radio. To make sure these people were at least aware that this programming was going to happen, we did mailings to our governor, and to state and federal legislators before each call-in show. We also sent information to all the primary care centers, health departments, and other state agencies that had a role in health care and welfare policy. We wanted to reach people who were in positions to make laws and regulations."

Sound Partners' director Beth Mastin says, "WVPN realized that they weren't reaching the people down in the hollers with their content and storytelling, but still found a way to make it work. They relied on the fact that Charleston, although it's the state capital, is still a pretty small town, and all the policy makers are there when the legislature is in session."

Pettey and the producer/reporter Susan Leffler organized four listener call-in programs on the subjects of welfare reform, rural health care, women's health care, and transportation, plus 26 three-minute features, each of which was a personal story of how a lack of access to health care had affected a family. WVPN broadcast Leffler's features during commuter drive times, catching lawmakers and government officials in their cars on the way to work.

"We had no illusions about reaching people on welfare with our broadcasts," Leffler says. "But with our series, the families who were dealing firsthand with the consequences of welfare reform got to tell their stories on the radio. I relied on WVPN's grass-roots outreach partners, such as Sister Brendan Conlon's

Christian Help Center, to identify people whose stories we could put on the air. They helped me get to them and win their confidence, but it was difficult. Sometimes, after making an appointment and driving two hours out of Charleston to talk with a family, I'd find them not at home. Often, I'd have to make two or three trips for the same three-minute segment. The outreach partners explained why that happened, and counseled me to be patient but persistent. For the first time, I grasped what it meant to have no telephone and no transportation."

Leffler's series aired from July through December, 1998. Early in 1999, a federal court ruled that children's SSI benefits were not to be counted as income in determining welfare eligibility. On March 13 of that year, the West Virginia legislature unanimously voted to restore welfare benefits to those who had been cut off under the SSI regulation. Although WVPN was not the only media outlet discussing the issue, advocates for low-income households credited *Health Care at the Crossroads* with focusing public debate and with being a major contributor to the policy reversal.

Leffler herself was pleased that her reporting had an impact, but she insists that she did not begin with the goal of reversing state welfare policy. "Listener call-ins and stories did not set out to promote a particular point of view," she says. "The series acted as a conduit between those whose health care was affected by welfare reform, the officials who were making policy, and the public who elected the officials."

~~ Promoting Civic Journalism

Whether this kind of reporting is viewed as civic journalism or advocacy depends on one's orientation. "Civic journalism is a way to do reporting that is more of a dialogue than a monologue," says Sound Partners director Beth Mastin, "and for some journalists, that's a sacrilege. Reporting to them by definition means that it's going in one direction."

"A number of the larger stations had concerns about blurring the lines between journalism and outreach to the community," says Sound Partners director Mark Sachs. "The issues centered on getting involved in the community instead of just reporting."

"At WVPN, the allegation that I had slipped into advocacy didn't really come during the course of the first round broadcasts," says Susan Leffler. "Interestingly, however, one of our former corporate partners later mentioned to the station general manager that he didn't feel our coverage in round 1 was 'objective.' Although he was a partner in the Sound Partners program, he never brought this up at meetings, but chose to save his criticism until after the fact. We also heard after the grant was over that the some of the department heads in the West Virginia Department of Health and Human Resources, who were responsible for welfare reform, weren't happy with our approach."

Sound Partners purposely did not define the working relationship between the radio stations and the partners, believing that the manner in which stations and partners came together to meet the goals of the program was one way to see civic journalism at work. Because civic journalism is a term which has no single meaning, various pairings of grantees forged their own definitions as they proceeded through the Sound Partners program.

—— Program Assessments

The impact of round 1 of the Sound Partners program was examined by four different studies: one by O'Neal-Hobbs Associates, another by the Cosmos Corporation, a third by Sharon Griggins, and the last by Livingston Associates.[2] The studies mainly relied on self-assessments of the projects by the staff of the radio stations and collaborating community organizations. The question of how to measure success arose. "One possible area of concern is evaluating the project using measurable data. Documenting success is difficult because of the nature of radio," wrote Tom Livingston of Livingston Associates in *Sound Partners Assessment*. "Success benchmarks and indicators were not established for first round Sound Partners grantees," wrote Loretta Hobbs in her report. "Consequently, stations identified as successes a broad range of factors."

Participants in the studies generally reported that their projects were successful, often in ways that were not anticipated at the outset of the program. "Sound Partners grants changed the way that stations gathered and reported the news," wrote Sharon Griggins in her report, *Sound Partners Lessons Learned Conference*. "The projects brought new voices to the radio. The Sound Partners grant changed the way participants and their organization viewed themselves and their communities."

"Several grantees affirmed that their listenership increased," wrote Loretta Hobbs in *Sound Partners for Community Health First Round Grantee Assessment*. "Others indicated their off-air town hall approach yielded fewer listeners, but significantly improved the quality and depth of community education and interaction. Some stations won awards, and one raised an additional $200,000 from another funder to continue broadcasting after the Sound Partners grant ended."

—— Round 2 and Beyond

It is too early in the round 2 grant cycle to assess the programs of new recipients. A number of returning grantees, however, have a very clear picture of how they are going to proceed. In general the approach is 'less is more.' "For round 2, we're going to be a little more realistic," says Joan Buffington of KVMR. "We're cutting the number of on-air programs in half and going bi-weekly. However, we're going to do what we had hoped to do in round 1, which is to produce some really well thought out longer pieces. This second round will have two stages. The bi-weekly program will provide the fuel, the raw material for two to four produced pieces, which will each be an hour long. We're going to take the raw material and use the nuggets of that to make some very powerful programming which can be used, not only in this community, but in other rural communities that are dealing with the same issues of gentrification, and how you pay for all the incredible costs of aging and chronic illness."

"For round 2, Leslie Rich of the Mendocino County Youth Project is going to play a much bigger role," says Jill Hannum of KZYX&Z. "She has written an awareness of lessons learned into the round 2 grant. We are going to streamline the program and focus on just two schools that have some geographic proximity to one another, so that the young people from those two schools can interact with each other as part of the project. We chose the two schools that have the most committed peer counseling advisors. In round 1, we found that without the advisor being committed to the project, the students did not want to become part of it either. We're also going to make the project more integrated with the classes."

"I'm working to identify teachers in the high schools who will make listening to the show an assignment for their students," says Leslie Rich. "We're also going to drop the prerecorded teen diary, which was very time-consuming to produce for both the peer counselors and radio station personnel."

"The kids will have on-air guests who will be people whose decisionmaking powers have some kind of impact on young people's lives," continues Hannum. "The idea would be to set it up so that the peer counselors can do research on a topic like Juvenile Hall, then bring someone like the sheriff or a probation officer on the show, and engage them in conversation to a point where the young people can feel as if they can have some impact in the community and get their voices heard. The show airs on Sunday night, which is a prime spot. We hope that in the second round we can really build this into something. We built a good audience in round 1, and people really appreciate the program, but it hasn't really had an impact yet on the community. We want to have the county supervisors say, "Well, this problem was brought to light on this radio show and now we're getting pressure from teens all over the county."

Sound Partners national staff will be working to deal with one inequality built into the program: it is the radio stations, not the stations and their community partners jointly, who receive the funding. "At the Lessons Learned Conference, held in 1999, some of the outreach partners told me that there was a really unequal power relationship in the program," continues Sachs. "Aside from the money, a number of partners felt that they were just there to fulfill the outreach provisions of the grant. In round 2, one of the things I'm going to do differently is to talk to stations on an ongoing basis, especially early in the program, to see if they have any issues with their partners, and how we can get them to work together on a more collaborative basis."

However Sound Partners evolves in round 2, the program has already shown itself to be an example of the philosophy that William Benton gave to the trustees of his foundation: "Favor those things which seem risky, unorthodox, hazardous, and even unlikely to succeed—but which, with success, offer more than ordinary promise and in some cases very exceptional promise."

Notes

1. V. Weisfeld. "The Foundation's Radio and Television Grants, 1987–1997." In S. L. Isaacs and J. R. Knickman (eds.), *To Improve Health and Health Care 1998-1999: The Robert Wood Johnson Foundation Anthology.* San Francisco: Jossey-Bass, 1998, provides a comprehensive review of the Foundation's work with National Public Radio and other radio and television broadcasting.

2. O'Neal-Hobbs Associates. *Sound Partners for Community Health First Round Grantee Assessment,* April 7, 2000; Cosmos. *Sound Partners for Community Health Final Evaluation Report,* February, 2000; S. Griggins, *Sound Partners Lessons Learned Conference,* May, 1999; Livingston Associates. *Sound Partners Assessment,* September 15, 1999.

꧁

Exhibit 7.1. Sound Partners for Community Health Grantees.

Round 1

Impact of Welfare Reform on Access to Health Care

Grantee	Location	Partner
WJAB-FM	Normal, Alabama	Alabama Cooperative Extension
KNAU-FM	Flagstaff, Arizona	*Daily Sun* newspaper and Institute for Native Americans at Northern Arizona University
KVMR-FM	Nevada City, California	Nevada County Department of Human Services and Foundation of Resources for Equality and Employment for the Disabled
KQED-FM	San Francisco, California	Homeless Prenatal Project of San Francisco
WVPE-FM	Elkhart, Indiana	Elkhart General Hospital; Saint Joseph's Medical Center; PARTNERS Health Plan; and Memorial Health system
WMMT-FM	Whitesburg, Kentucky	Center for Rural Health at University of Kentucky; Kentuckians for the Commonwealth; Appalachian Research and Defense Fund; Office of Kentucky Legal Service Programs; Kentucky Welfare Reform Coalition; Kentucky Youth Advocates; and National Health Law
KFAI-FM	Minneapolis, Minnesota	Neighborhood Health Care Network
KDNA-FM	Granger, Washington	Yakima Valley Farm Workers Clinic and Department of Social and Health Services
KWSU-AM	Pullman, Washington	Washington's Department of Social and Health Services; Women's Resource Center at Columbia Basin College; Human Services Coalition in Tri-Cities, Washington; Opportunity Council in Bellingham, Washington; Idaho's Department of Health and Welfare; and Clallum County Health Department
WVPN-FM	Charleston, West Virginia	Robert C. Byrd Health Sciences Center

JP

Exhibit 7.1.   Sound Partners for Community Health Grantees, *continued.*

Providing Health Care to Children

Grantee	Location	Partner
KBRW-AM	Anchorage, Alaska	Women, Infant, and Children's nutrition program; Alaska Native Health Board; and Chugachmuit
KCAW-FM	Sitka, Alaska	Southeast Alaska Regional Health Consortium; Center for Community/Infant Learning Program; and State of Alaska Public Health Nurse
KHDC-FM	Salinas, California	Head Start
WDET-FM	Detroit, Michigan	William Beaumont Hospital
KCUR-FM	Kansas City, Missouri	Partnership for Children
KXCV-FM	Maryville, Missouri	Northwest Missouri Regional Council of Government; Community Solution for Rural Health of Nodaway County; Heartland Regional Community Foundation; and Center for Applied Research at Northwest Missouri State University
WUNM-FM	Albuquerque, New Mexico	South West Organizing Project
WAMC-FM	Albany, New York	Albany County Health Department; Albany Medical Center; Kaiser Permanente; Saint Peter's Hospital; and Whitney M. Young, Jr. Health Center
KSTX-FM	San Antonio, Texas	San Antonio Metropolitan Health District

New Approaches to Curtailing Youth Substance Abuse

Grantee	Location	Partner
KIYU-AM	Galena, Alaska	Yukon-Koyukuk Mental Health
KZYX&Z-FM	Philo, California	Mendocino County Youth Project
WKMS-FM	Murray, Kentucky	Regional Prevention Center

℘

Exhibit 7.1. Sound Partners for Community Health Grantees, *continued.*

New Approaches to Curtailing Youth Substance Abuse, continued

Grantee	Location	Partner
WSLU-FM	Canton, New York	Saint Joseph's Rehabilitation Center
WBAI-FM	New York, New York	Global Kids
WAER-FM	Syracuse, New York	Syracuse Onondaga Drug and Alcohol Abuse Commission
WRTU-FM	San Juan, Puerto Rico	Center for Rehabilitation through the Arts
WMRA-FM	Harrisonburg, Virginia	VaLiance Health Partners and Search Institute of Minneapolis
WOJB-FM	Hayward, Wisconsin	Lac Courte Oreille Tribe

Health Care Decision Making at the End of Life

Grantee	Location	Partner
KUAF-FM	Fayetteville, Arkansas	Washington Regional Medical Center Hospice
KLRE-FM and KUAR-FM	Little Rock, Arkansas	University of Arkansas for Medical Sciences
KGNU-FM	Boulder, Colorado	Hospice of Boulder County
WBST-FM	Muncie, Indiana	Center for Gerontology at Fisher Institute for Wellness at Ball State University
KUFM-FM	Missoula, Montana	Missoula Demonstration Project
KUCV-FM	Lincoln, Nebraska	Alzheimer's Association
WSKG-FM	Binghamton, New York	United Health Services; Center for Healthy Aging; Four County Library System; and Health Science Center Clinical Campus at State University of New York at Binghamton

જ્ર

Exhibit 7.1. Sound Partners for Community Health Grantees, *continued.*

Round 2

Maintaining the Health Care Safety Net

Grantee	Location	Partner
WCBU-FM	Peoria, Illinois	Methodist Medical Center
WUOM-FM	Ann Arbor, Michigan	Michigan Public Health Institute and Center for Advancing Community Health
WNMU-FM	Marquette, Michigan	Western Upper Peninsula District Health Department
KZUM-FM	Lincoln, Nebraska	Lincoln Interfaith Council and Lincoln Public Schools
WRNI-FM	Barrington, Rhode Island	Rhode Island Foundation
KDNA-FM	Granger, Washington	Yakima Valley Farm Workers Clinic and Providence Health System of Central Washington
WVPN-FM	Charleston, West Virginia	West Virginia Community Voices Partnership; West Virginia Economic Justice Project; Office of Community and Rural Health; West Virginia Health Rights; Christian Help; and West Virginia Healthy Kids Coalition

Providing Health Care for Children

Grantee	Location	Partner
KCAW-FM	Sitka, Alaska	South East Alaska Regional Health Consortium; Islands Counseling Services; and Sitka Public Health Nursing
WUFT-FM	Gainesville, Florida	Child Care Resources
WMPG-FM	Portland, Maine	City of Portland Public Health Division
KFAI-FM	Minneapolis, Minnesota	Neighborhood Health Care Network and La Prensa

Exhibit 7.1. Sound Partners for Community Health Grantees, *continued.*

Providing Health Care for Young Children, continued

Grantee	Location	Partner
KWMU-FM	St. Louis, Missouri	St. Louis Children's Hospital
KCEP-FM	Las Vegas, Nevada	Clark County SAFE KIDS Coalition; University Medical Center's Burn Unit; Alisa Ann Ruch Burn Foundation; Clark County Fire Department; Clark County Health District; and Lions Club

New Approaches to Curtailing Youth Substance Abuse

Grantee	Location	Partner
KUAC-FM	Fairbanks, Alaska	Fairbanks Native Association
WVAS-FM	Montgomery, Alabama	Baptist Hospital System and Alabama Cooperative Extension System
KUAF-FM	Fayetteville, Arkansas	Art Experience of Fayetteville
KZYX-FM and KZYZ-FM	Philo, California	Mendocino County Youth Project
WRTE-FM	Chicago, Illinois	Illinois Masonic Medical Center
WFPK-FM and WFPL-FM	Louisville, Kentucky	University of Louisville Hospital and Kentucky Cancer Program
WBAI-FM	New York, New York	Global Kids and Center for Alcohol and Substance Abuse at Columbia University
WDIY-FM	Bethlehem, Pennsylvania	ALERT Partnership
KSER-FM	Lynnwood, Washington	Snohomish Health District; Everett AquaSox Baseball Club; Everett Alternatives High School; Everett Community College; and Everett YMCA
WVMR-AM	Dunmore, West Virginia	High Rocks Academy

ॐ

Exhibit 7.1. Sound Partners for Community Health Grantees, *continued*.

Health Care Decision Making at the End of Life

Grantee	Location	Partner
WLRN-FM	Miami, Florida	Hospice Care of Broward County
WKMS-FM	Murray, Kentucky	Department of Nursing at Murray State University
WNED-FM	Buffalo, New York	Center for Hospice and Palliative Care; Graduate School of Education at University of Buffalo; Erie County Bar Association; and WNED-TV
KOPB-FM and KOAC-AM	Portland, Oregon	Oregon Health Forum; Oregon Hospice Association; and Oregon Health Sciences University
WUWM-FM	Milwaukee, Wisconsin	Medical College of Wisconsin

Caring for the Aging and Chronically Ill

Grantee	Location	Partner
KVMR-FM	Nevada City, California	Foundation of Resources for Equality and Employment for the Disabled
KXJZ-FM and KXPR-FM	Sacramento, California	Gerontology Department at California State University at Sacramento
KBBF-FM	Santa Rosa, California	Sonoma County Area Agency on Aging and Sonoma County Human Services Department
WPKT-FM	Hartford, Connecticut	School of Nursing at Yale University
WDCB-FM	Glen Ellyn, Illinois	DuPage County Health Department and DuPage County Human Services

A Look Back

CHAPTER EIGHT

~~ The Regionalized Perinatal Care Program

Marguerite Y. Holloway

Editors' Introduction

In this chapter, Marguerite Holloway, a contributing editor for *Scientific American* and an adjunct professor of journalism at Columbia University, looks back at the efforts of The Robert Wood Johnson Foundation in the 1970s and 1980s to encourage the regionalization of perinatal services—the care delivered to mother and child shortly before and after birth. The development of high-technology care delivered in neonatal intensive care units made it possible to save the lives of low-birthweight babies who previously might have died. But not every hospital could have the sophisticated equipment and specialized staff to care for the small percentage of infants requiring intensive care. It made sense, in the eyes of many maternal and child health experts, to organize services along geographic lines in a pyramid fashion. Pregnant women at risk of delivering a low-birthweight baby would be identified early and transferred up the pyramid to a hospital capable of offering the care necessary. At the top of the pyramid would be a level III hospital—often at an academic medical center—that would treat the most needy newborns in a high-tech neonatal intensive care unit.

Building on regional arrangements to provide care for specific illnesses in the United States and reports of success with regional perinatal care networks in Canada, the Foundation funded an eight-site demonstration program—the Regionalized Perinatal Care Program—to determine whether the regionalization of perinatal services would work on a large scale and with heterogeneous populations.

As Holloway observes, the path has been rocky, and long-term successes have been elusive. While the grantees funded under the program—as well as the comparison sites—made progress toward regionalization and lowering neonatal mortality rates, these achievements often evaporated after funding ended. And from the mid-1980s on, managed care organizations seemed to be directing people to their own networks rather than to networks built along geographical lines.

What is most disturbing about the story is that while infant and neonatal mortality rates have declined over the past 30 years, severe racial, economic, and class differences in low-birthweight, preterm delivery, and infant mortality rates persist. Even though this is a retrospective review of past programs, the hope is that it will stimulate new thinking on strategies that the nation can pursue to improve perinatal care.

Two or three times a week, David A. Yost, clinical director at the Whiteriver Indian Hospital in Arizona, transfers a pregnant patient by plane or helicopter to the Good Samaritan Hospital in Phoenix, some 200 miles away. "It is for a wide variety of causes: from a teenage mother with early labor, or twins, to complications from trauma or diabetes," he says. "We have a lot of preeclampsia, infectious disease, and diabetes, and a lot of that leads to prematurity. We also have a lot of alcoholism, fetal alcohol syndrome, and trauma from car accidents in our pregnant patients." Because the Whiteriver Indian Hospital, which is on the Fort Apache Indian Reservation in the eastern part of the state, does not have a neonatal intensive care unit, or NICU, these women and their babies—90 percent of whom are covered by Medicaid—would be in danger unless they could be quickly moved to a fully equipped center.

To try to ensure that Yost and his counterparts in remote areas throughout Arizona have access to university hospitals and large medical centers with perinatologists or NICUs, the state maintains a voluntary perinatal referral and transportation network called the Arizona Perinatal Trust. "The system works," Yost says—except, he adds, sometimes in the winter. "This is a high area and there is lots of snow and in bad weather, if you can't get the airplane on the ground or the patient out the door, you are stuck. But that is just part of living rural."

—— The Emergence of Perinatal Care

The Arizona Perinatal Trust arose out of a program funded by The Robert Wood Johnson Foundation in the 1970s to regionalize administration of perinatal care—that is, the care offered to a mother and child just before and just after birth. Perinatal intensive care is a relatively young field, one that emerged in the 1950s and 1960s as a result of technological innovations. The development of ventilation machines and better incubators led to the creation of modern NICUs. In addition, ultrasound, amniocentesis, electronic monitoring of fetal circulation during labor, and various biochemical tests could reveal whether the baby's growth was slow, whether it was in distress, and whether it would be able to breathe on its own. Armed with this

◎

Table 8.1.   Glossary of Terms.

Term	Definition
Neonatal	Pertaining to the period of time from birth to the fourth week after birth.
Perinatal	Pertaining to the period of time from the completion of 28 weeks of gestation to 1–4 weeks after birth.
Post-neonatal	Pertaining to the period from the fourth week after birth to the end of the first year.
Preterm	An infant born between the twentieth week and the thirty-eighth week of gestation (134 to 266 days). Normal gestation is approximately forty weeks.
Low Birthweight (LBW)	Birthweight of less than 2,500 grams (5 lbs., 8 oz.).
Very Low Birthweight (VLBW)	Birthweight of less than 1,500 grams (3 lbs., 4 oz.).
Mortality	The death rate, usually reported as the ratio of number of deaths to a given population.
Morbidity	The disease rate, usually reported as the ratio of persons with a particular disease to a given population.
Infant Mortality	The rate of death that occurs between birth and the end of the first year, which includes both the neonatal and post-neonatal periods.

Sources: Thomas, C. L., *Taber's Cyclopedic Medical Dictionary*. Philadelphia: F.A. Davis Company, 1973. *National Vital Statistics Report*, April 29, 1999, volume 47, number 18. UNICEF (United Nations Children's Fund), *The State of the World's Children 2000*. New York: Oxford University Press, 2000.

detailed information and new technology, pediatricians were able to identify high-risk mothers and infants and make a difference.

The results of these interventions were dramatic. Reports from several researchers showed that the interventions had a powerful effect on mortality and morbidity. Working in the 1960s in Quebec, Mary Ellen Avery, currently at Harvard University, showed that state-of-the-art intervention reduced the incidence of neurosensory damage—such as mental retardation, cerebral palsy, and epilepsy—in very low-birthweight babies from between 75 and 70 percent to between 20 and 15 percent.[1] A 1973 paper in the *British Medical Journal* reported that among 500 high-risk births at St. Thomas' Hospital in London there were no cases of mental retardation if modern methods were used; normally, 10 such cases would have been expected.[2] Reports from various other areas—including Arizona and Ohio—also pointed to increased survival when newborns were given access to special care.[3]

But "the study that had really excited the attention of pediatricians and pediatric nurses was a report from Toronto," recalls Kenneth G. Johnson, a physician who directed the Foundation-funded Regionalized Perinatal Care Program. "There were two very good perinatal networks, and they showed that it was just the access to specialized care that was needed."

Thus by the late 1960s and the early 1970s, it had become clear to the medical community that neonatal mortality could be dramatically curtailed if patients had access to specialists, to newly proven technologies, and to NICUs. These things were in short supply at the time, however, and it seemed apparent to many people practicing and studying perinatal care that one cost-effective way to improve access for parents in need would be to establish regional networks. In such systems, hospitals with different capabilities would coordinate care. A rural or community health center such as Whiteriver Indian Hospital could transfer a mother whom doctors deemed to be at high risk for premature delivery to a facility that had the requisite NICU. Ideally, such regional organizations would permit every mother and infant access to the right level of care. And they would contain medical costs, because hospitals would not have to build NICUs or recruit perinatologists if they were part of a network with a center that was already so equipped.

The medical community responded quickly. In 1971, the American Medical Association issued a statement on the benefits of regionalized perinatal care. The following year, experts from the American Academy of Pediatrics, the American Academy of Family Physicians, the American Medical Association, the American College of Obstetricians and Gynecologists, and the March of Dimes Birth Defects Foundation (then the National Foundation-March of Dimes) met in San Francisco to discuss regionalization. The participants formed a Committee on Perinatal Health, and agreed that implementing systems of community or regionalized perinatal care was imperative. Other changes soon followed: the American College of Obstetricians and Gynecologists formed a maternal-fetal medicine sub-board in

1972; the American Academy of Pediatrics established a specialization in neonatology-perinatology in 1973, and in 1975, neonatal-perinatal medicine became a board-certified subspecialty.

The growing consensus of the medical community was gathered in what has come to be called by many the bible of perinatal care: "Toward Improving the Outcome of Pregnancy: Recommendations for the Regional Development of Maternal and Perinatal Health Services." Published in 1976 by the March of Dimes Birth Defects Foundation, the report outlined the need for a consistent system to screen mothers and infants to determine who was at high risk; it defined levels, or types, of hospitals and the care that was appropriate to receive at each; it emphasized the need for a uniform data system, and it stressed the importance of education and outreach within the medical community.

⎯ The Regional Perinatal Network

Regionalization of care was not a new idea. Certain areas in the United States had coordinated aspects of their medical services during the 1940s. And in 1965, the federal government had authorized the funding of so called Regional Medical Programs to increase the access of heart disease, stroke, and cancer patients to new equipment and procedures.[4] But opposition by elements of the medical profession was fierce, and the results of these efforts were ambiguous. For the most part regionalization remained untested. "At that time, there was a lot of disbelief," recalls George A. Little, a neonatologist at the Dartmouth-Hitchcock Medical Center in Lebanon, New Hampshire. "People needed to be convinced about applying care in a regional fashion. It was not the way that acute care was practiced."

As the groundswell of national interest was emerging, The Robert Wood Johnson Foundation began to explore whether regional perinatal networks were indeed feasible, whether they could reduce neonatal mortality, and if so, whether decreasing mortality resulted in an increase in developmental or other problems as low-birthweight babies survived. One of the principle catalysts for the Foundation's involvement was Irwin R. Merkatz, now chairman of the Department of Obstetrics and Gynecology at the Albert Einstein College of Medicine of Yeshiva University in the Bronx, and then at Case Western Reserve University in Cleveland, Ohio. During 1972 and 1973, Merkatz spoke with Walsh McDermott, special adviser to the Foundation, and David E. Rogers, president of the Foundation, about the importance of undertaking a perinatal demonstration project. It was an opportunity, they agreed, to do widely what had been shown in only a few places as workable. Within the Foundation, McDermott developed the idea of funding a demonstration to test the feasibility of establishing regional perinatal networks.

In 1974, the Foundation issued a Call for Proposals. "The nuts and bolts were pretty straightforward," Johnson says. "All the hospitals in a defined area had to come together. And the level I, level II, and level III hospitals had to agree to follow a protocol and the use of a systematic problem-oriented risk assessment system." Although definitions can vary by state, in general, level I refers to a facility that can care for normal or mildly ill newborns; level IIs can deal with infants at moderate risk; and level IIIs have NICUs and can tend to very sick infants. The networks also had to establish a system of referral and maternal or infant transportation, and had to conduct outreach and education. In other words, the project would test the major elements that were being discussed in the perinatal community—and that came to be enumerated in the March of Dimes report.

After reviewing 34 applications, the Foundation selected eight sites (see Table 8.2 on page 182) and awarded $17.6 million in grants between 1975 and 1979. The grantees were chosen because they were geographically, socially, and economically diverse: the state of Arizona, Cleveland, Dallas County in Texas, three contiguous areas in Los Angeles, Manhattan's Upper West Side, and a 15-county area around Syracuse, New York. The thought was that if the demonstrations of regional networks worked in these very different places, they would serve as models for similar regions elsewhere.

Although there were vast differences among the sites, many of the challenges they faced in implementing networks were the same. According to Johnson, friction between the community hospitals and the level IIIs sometimes became debilitating. Doctors often did not want to lose their patients; for some, it was simply a matter of ego. In other places, reimbursement for transportation expenses became a source of conflict.

Record keeping also proved to be a challenge. Merkatz and Calvin J. Hobel, who served as director of the Los Angeles South Bay Regional Perinatal Project, designed a record-keeping system called The Problem Oriented Perinatal Risk Assessment System, or POPRAS. POPRAS enabled every participating institution and health care provider to

Table 8.2. The Eight Sites in the Regionalized Perinatal Care Program.

Grantee Name	Location	Years	Funding Amount
Arizona Medical Association Foundation	Phoenix, Arizona	1975–1982	$2,200,000
Case Western Reserve University School of Medicine	Cleveland, Ohio	1975–1981	2,225,000
Charles R. Drew University of Medicine and Science	Los Angeles, California	1975–1982	2,200,000
Columbia University College of Physicians and Surgeons	New York, New York	1975–1982	2,199,925
Health Science Center, State University of New York at Syracuse	Syracuse, New York	1975–1982	2,176,351
Health Science Center, University of Texas at Dallas	Dallas, Texas	1975–1981	2,200,000
Professional Staff Association of Los Angeles County at Harbor General Hospital	Torrance, California	1975–1981	2,200,000
University of Southern California School of Medicine	Los Angeles, California	1975–1983	2,198,721

assess and record risk factors, medical information, and care in a consistent way—a crucial need since patients were going to be moving around. All pregnant women were to be evaluated at least twice during the prenatal period, again during delivery, and after birth. "It was a kind of sea change in the whole movement," comments David E. Gagnon, president of the National Perinatal Information Center in Providence, Rhode Island. "POPRAS was an extensive risk identification system that many later imitated."

Although POPRAS was designed to be the centerpiece of the program—Kenneth Johnson recalls that 60 to 70 percent of the grant money was spent on this aspect—many of the participants had trouble initially setting up the system. It was adopted by four of the sites. Moreover, for some physicians, the uniform risk identification system was threatening. They were worried that if a mother's risk score was high and they decided not to transfer her, they would be vulnerable to malpractice action. "It was very difficult to get the hospitals and the physicians used to the assessment system," Johnson says. "They just hated it." Other health care workers were concerned about the privacy of their patients, an issue that still resonates today. Johnson recalls that the program attempted to deal with both concerns—by getting informed consent from the patients and by showing that the scoring system was not perfect and that physician judgment remained an important part of risk assessment.

Despite the kinks, most participants reported that the networks functioned well,[5] and that regional involvement was between 80 and 100 percent except in some of the rural areas, such as Arizona and upstate New York, where facilities were far-flung and only about 60 to 70 percent of the hospitals in the region became partners.[6] It was also apparent that the identification of high-risk mothers led to many more instances of maternal, as opposed to neonatal, transfer—a sign of success to perinatologists. "There was a shift from the emphasis on the transport of the infant into the referral center to the transport of the mother prior to birth," Gagnon says. "The whole idea was that the best transport unit is the mother's uterus."

Wendy Reynolds of Cleveland agrees that this approach probably saved one of her children. In July of 1977, her daughter, Alicia, was born two-and-a-half months early. "She was in a hurry. She was going to come whether we wanted her to or not," Reynolds says. "It was fairly early in the morning, around 1 A.M., and I woke up because I had to sneeze, and when I sneezed, my water broke. My husband was home, thank God, and he took me to the hospital then. And they monitored me for a little while. They were trying to see if I was really going to give birth. And when they determined I was, they transferred me." Reynolds was moved by ambulance from a level I hospital to a nearby university hospital. Twelve hours later, Reynolds gave birth to Alicia, who stayed in the NICU until she was out of danger. She finally came home in September—almost exactly to the day that she was originally due.

⟶ Evaluating the Program

Once the Regionalized Perinatal Care Program ended, the next step was to quantify the project's effects, and, in particular, to address a concern that had been raised at the outset. "The Foundation had many critics at the time we announced the program," Johnson notes. "One serious criticism was that we would reduce mortality, but that these kids would have other problems and that we were not addressing root causes."

In 1980, the Foundation awarded $2.8 million to three researchers for a two-year evaluation of the project. Marie C. McCormick, who was then at Johns Hopkins University (and who is currently a professor of pediatrics at Harvard University) and her colleagues Sam Shapiro and Barbara H. Starfield set out to determine whether infant mortality had fallen at the eight sites and, if so, whether that decline was due to increased survival of high-risk infants or to a decrease in the number of low-birthweight babies, to regionalization, or to other factors. Their review ultimately appeared in *The Journal of the American Medical Association* in 1985.

The team found that so much had been happening to improve perinatal health nationally that it was hard to see any effect at the eight projects that differed from effects that were occurring in the rest of the country. Neonatal mortality rates had fallen not only at the eight sites but also in the comparison regions: an 18-county area around Albany; six health districts in Brooklyn, New York; a six-county area around Buffalo, New York; Harris and Tarrant counties in Texas; an 11-county area around Rochester, New York; San Diego county; and, finally, Wayne County, Michigan. Between 1974 or 1975 and 1978 or 1979, neonatal mortality in the funded areas fell an average of 19 percent, while it dropped by 25 percent in the comparison areas.[7] The evaluators attributed two-thirds of the decline to the increased survival of low-birthweight babies. This increased survival was due, in turn, the authors noted, to the early identification of at-risk mothers and to the increased delivery of high-risk infants in tertiary centers—that is, level IIIs. Regionalization had clearly shifted the location of delivery: by the end of the decade, 50 percent of low-birthweight babies and 60 percent of very low-birthweight babies were being delivered in level III centers in the foundation-funded areas. And, according to Johnson, whereas before the program about 90 percent of the transfers were made after the baby was born, about half of the transfers were now made before birth.

Again, in the comparison areas, the same shift had occurred. "The centralization of high-risk deliveries appeared so widespread that the special effect of the RWJF program could not be detected," the authors concluded. They noted that although the degree of change in the comparison areas could not have been predicted at the start of the program, the March of Dimes recommendations published in 1976 and the publicity given to the Foundation's program "may have encouraged regionalization in the absence of specific funding."

The evaluation also addressed the issue of morbidity. The study found that, at one year of age, there was no increased incidence of congenital anomalies or developmental delays among low-birthweight babies. Developmental delays and congenital anomalies actually decreased by about 15 percent, and most dramatically in the very low-birthweight group: by about 22 percent.[8] This was not, however, the final word on low birthweight and child health.

The Regionalized Perinatal Care Program was followed by a study of long-term development in babies of varying weights, to see how they fared at 8 to 10 years of age, and by a study of the effects of educational intervention.[9] Marie McCormick, the leader of the evaluation team, and several colleagues continued to monitor some of the babies born at the eight sites. They—and other researchers—found that low-birthweight babies are at increased risk for behavioral and learning disorders, asthma, and other health problems, and that the incidence and severity of those problems increases as birthweight falls.[10]

The findings from the evaluation of the Regionalized Perinatal Care Program indicated that a national trend toward regionalization of perinatal services had emerged, to the degree that the Foundation-funded sites represented, as L. Joseph Butterworth, a pediatrician at the Children's Hospital in Denver, Colorado, remarked many years ago, "eight large boulders in a landslide."[11] Yet the Foundation's role was not insignificant, "What the Foundation did was, in a sense, to support something that was emerging at a critical time," says the National Perinatal Information Center's Gagnon. "They tested it and drew attention to it."

—— The Regional Networks After the Program

Over the years, the eight Foundation-funded networks each went their separate ways. Some fell apart—including the networks in Los Angeles and Dallas County, Texas[12]—while the others evolved. Arizona, for its part, took the money left over from its grant, combined it with funds from Samaritan Health Services and St. Joseph's Hospital in Phoenix, and in 1980 established the Arizona Perinatal Regional System, Inc. This body oversees a voluntary certification system for participants: the Arizona Perinatal Trust, which David Yost is part of today. Cleveland and New York, in turn, received state support to continue the networks in some form.

But Arizona and New York were not able to keep the records system in place. "One of the big problems we had was that The Robert Wood Johnson Foundation had funded a huge statewide data system," says Deb Christian, executive director of the Arizona Perinatal Trust. "After the program ended, entry of that data stopped." Christian notes that the lack of a continuing record system hinders the effectiveness of the network. The same holds true in New York, where the state Department of Health is just starting a statewide Perinatal Data System.

A dearth of data is something that many perinatologists around the country are decrying, particularly as they struggle to understand the persistence of preterm delivery, low birthweight, and racial differences in neonatal mortality. "A major barrier to monitoring neonatal intensive care on a large scale is the lack of adequate data sources," note Jeffrey D. Horbar and Jerold F. Lucey in "The Future of Children," a report published in 1995 by the David and Lucile Packard Foundation.[13]

The fact that perinatologists are still calling for a uniform perinatal data system angers Irwin Merkatz, who argues that POPRAS should have been maintained and extended—with Foundation money. "There were many systems that needed not only initial investment but continued investment," he says. In addition, Merkatz believes that the Foundation should have worked to get states more focused on maternal and child health, to leverage the experience of the networks while it was still hot. "My view is that the Foundation was uniquely placed to build upon their success and to make the next level of investment to keep that moving forward," he says. "Now here we are in 1999, and we are still lacking a comprehensive system of maternal and child health."

Within the Foundation, there is some consensus that there should have been more follow-up for the Regionalized Perinatal Care Program. "The prevailing philosophy at that time was that we would absolutely not do follow-up grants," says Frank Karel, vice-president for communications at The Robert Wood Johnson Foundation. "We would plot out what was a reasonable trajectory and then it was on its own." Today, he says, the Foundation has seen the error of that rigidity; there is more openness to longer programs and to follow-on initiatives.

⎯⎯ The Rural Infant Care Program

Although the Foundation did not sustain its involvement with the eight regional perinatal networks, it did continue to examine perinatal health through a variety of programs, trying to identify gaps in the medical delivery system and to address infant mortality and morbidity. Between 1980 and 1985, the Foundation, under the Rural Infant Care Program, gave $8.3 million to 10 medical schools to work with state and local health departments in rural areas that were isolated, where poverty was high, and where residents had poor access to care. The project activities ranged from organizing meetings among physicians, hospital administrators, and public health department staff to expanding prenatal services and instituting regionalization of perinatal care. A later evaluation found that in funded areas neonatal mortality decreased by 2.6 per 1,000 births; among blacks, that figure was even higher: a reduction of 4.5 per 1,000.[14] Three groups of comparison areas that did not receive Foundation funding experienced no significant changes in neonatal mortality rates. The decrease in mortality was attributed to reduced mortality among low-birthweight babies—many more of whom were being born in tertiary centers. The incidence of low-birthweight deliveries remained the same, however.

The Rural Infant Care Program was intended to follow up on the insights gleaned during the Regionalized Perinatal Care Program. "We brought the same approach to the 10 states with excessive infant mortality," Kenneth Johnson says. "And there again we were able to form a partnership between a maternal and child health department in the state and the hospitals and the practitioners taking care of their patients."

⎯⎯ Regional Perinatal Services Today

The landslide to which the Foundation contributed eight boulders in the 1970s continued into the 1980s. In 1978, the Department of Health and Human Services issued guidelines mandating that neonatal and maternal obstetrics be planned on a regional model,[15] and by the end of the 1980s, 26 states had established referral systems or had guidelines for perinatal networks in place.[16]

Regional networks have been widely credited as one of the principle reasons for the rapid decline in neonatal mortality rates in the last several decades. (The other principal reason is the introduction in the late 1980s of surfactant replacement therapy, which reduced the incidence of lung disease in newborns.) Over the years, several studies have confirmed the value of transferring high-risk mothers and infants into level IIIs. For example, Nigel S. Paneth of Michigan State University found that mortality of low-birthweight babies was significantly higher in level I and level II centers than it was in level IIIs—in some areas, mortality decreased by one third to one half when the babies were tended to in tertiary centers.

Despite their recognized effectiveness, however, regional perinatal networks have begun to fall apart. They began to unravel in the 1980s, and the process continued with greater velocity in the 1990s. Two primary reasons explain this: first, the competition for patients that has developed between level II and level III hospitals and, second, the effect of managed care, which encourages the transfer of patients within the managed care company's network rather than within geographically constructed networks.

The first of these reasons stems, paradoxically, from the very recommendations the perinatal community made in the early 1970s. Because of the new programs in perinatology, a wealth of specialists began to hit the job market and, since the level IIIs were filled up, started working in level II hospitals. At about the same time, in the 1980s, the number of obstetrical malpractice suits rose, so more obstetricians started demanding that perinatologists or neonatologists be in attendance in their hospitals. Currently, these specialists appear to be in anything but short supply: by some estimates, there are 3,500 neonatal physicians. "I always incur a lot of rancor, because my sense is that we have about twice as many as we need or should have," says James Lemons, professor of pediatrics at Indiana University and chair of the American Academy of Pediatrics Committee on Fetus and Newborn.

In addition, hospitals began trying to attract a clientele in an increasingly competitive market, and having an NICU was one way to do this. Indeed, the proliferation of neonatal units has been stunning. In 1979, there were about 315 units in the United States; by 1997, there were 1,085.[17] And between 1983 and 1997, according to David Gagnon of the National Perinatal Information Center and his colleague Rachel M. Schwartz, the number of neonatal beds has grown from 6,893 to 11,908.[18] Gagnon estimates that there are twice as many beds as needed.

These changes have meant that level II hospitals increasingly want to hold on to their pregnant patients and newborns. The perinatologists, understandably, want to practice their craft; the hospitals want to get some return on their NICU or other neonatal investments. As a result, says George Little of the Dartmouth-Hitchcock Medical Center, "women with high-risk pregnancies may not be moved as quickly as they were in the past because of interest in maintaining these systems." The problem with this trend is that level IIs still may not always have the volume of patients needed to keep their practitioners as honed and skilled as they should be.

Some of the literature seems to support this conclusion. A recent study conducted in Missouri found that there had been a shift of deliveries into level IIs that had designated themselves perinatal centers, but that neonatal mortality in those centers remained twice that of the level IIIs.[19] Another study found the same thing in South Carolina: "Very low birthweight infants are more likely to survive if born in level III hospitals than in level I or level II facilities, with or without neonatologists."[20] And a report by Ciaran S. Phibbs of Stanford University and his colleagues concluded that "the rapid expansion of level II and level II+ NICUs in California in the 1980s has probably resulted in significantly higher risk-adjusted neonatal mortality than would have occurred if more of the care for high-risk deliveries had been concentrated in hospitals with level III NICUs."[21]

David Gagnon is not sure he agrees that the proliferation of level IIs inevitably leads to poorer care. "My own personal feeling is that that is not necessarily the case," he says. And he notes that the ability of community and level II hospitals to deal with high-risk infants is often comforting for mothers, who sometimes ended up far from their homes, families, and physicians when they were transferred—which was one of the criticisms of regional perinatal networks.[22] But, he adds, the proliferation "certainly cannot be justified on an economic basis." Gagnon suspects that the surplus of beds and specialists will lead to consolidation, which he is already seeing in places like Minnesota, where there used to be 10 NICUs in the state and there are now only four, concentrated in urban areas.

Another challenge comes from managed care, with its financial incentive to refer patients within its own managed care network rather than to a competing network. In some areas, hospitals that would have referred high-risk mothers to a nearby university center are instead holding on to their patients, hiring perinatologists and upgrading their facilities—many have gone to the multi-million dollar expense of building an NICU. Although definitive answers are not yet available, this situation worries some observers who fear that managed care is undermining the proven effectiveness of regional networks and in some cases may be jeopardizing infant health. 'There is a basic mismatch between managed care populations versus geographical populations," notes Bernard Guyer, a professor and chair of the Department of Population and Family Health Sciences at Johns Hopkins University. "From what I am seeing, managed care is changing the pattern of referral," adds Michigan State's Nigel Paneth. "Those patterns clearly have a lot to do with mortality."

⸺ What's Next for Regional Perinatal Networks

The crumbling of regional perinatal networks is occurring within a health system that continues to lag behind those of other developed countries. Although infant and maternal mortality have declined steadily since 1900—by more than 90 percent in total—America ranks 25th in the world in terms of infant mortality, with an average of 7.2 deaths per 1,000 live births in 1997.[23] By contrast, Japan has the lowest infant mortality rate, with 4 deaths per 1,000, and Sierra Leone has the highest, with 170 deaths, according to the United Nations.[24]

A closer look at the statistics reveals another disturbing trend as well—the persistence of a severe racial and economic gap in infant mortality rates despite the overall national decline. In 1997, 13.7 per 1,000 black infants died in the United States as opposed to 6 per 1,000 white infants.[25] In 1980, 22.2 per 1,000 black infants died compared to 10.9 per 1,000 white infants.[26] Neonatal mortality rates exhibit the same racial and economic gap.

In addition, neither the low-birthweight rate nor the preterm delivery rate has improved in America in the past 30 years.[27] Indeed, the rates in the past decade and a half have been increasing. Preterm deliveries increased from 9.4 per 1.000 in 1981 to 11.4 per 1,000 in 1997 for all newborns.[28] Likewise, low-birthweight newborns increased from 6.8 per 1,000 in 1981 to 7.5 per 1,000 in 1997.[29] Low-birthweight occurs in 7 percent of births—and those babies are 40 times as likely to die as are heavier babies. And, again, the incidence of low-birthweight and preterm delivery is about two times as high among African Americans as it is among whites.[30] Although African Americans are responsible for 17 percent of the country's births, they have 33 percent of low-birthweight babies and 38 percent of very low-birthweight babies.[31]

In 1998, for the first time in decades, the neonatal mortality rate did not fall,[32] but it is too early to tell whether this marks a decline in the quality of perinatal care, and if so, whether that decline has anything at all to do with the erosion of regional referral systems and perinatal networks. What does seem clear, however, is that the regionalized perinatal networks that emerged in the 1970s introduced the possibility of bringing maternal and child health into a unified system— and that this approach powerfully improved health.

Experts agree that even though the unified record-keeping model and the region-wide system of communication were never universally adopted, they are still relevant today: they offer a means of tracking risk and care in a way that could shed greater light on the persistent and poorly understood issues of preterm delivery, low birthweight, and racial differences. So it remains perplexing and upsetting to many observers—James Lemons and Irwin Merkatz among them—that by the end of the 1970s the country seemed ideally poised to build on the regional perinatal networks and to further improve and integrate maternal and child health care services, and that now, at the beginning of the twenty-first century, such a system is not in place. Given this, the strengths and failings of the Foundation's Regionalized Perinatal Care Program have particular resonance today. The program's accomplishments as well as its limitations—and, some would argue, its failings—suggest that a stronger national mechanism needs to be in place in order to better protect infant and maternal health.

Notes

1. Study cited by W. McDermott in *The Madonna Paper*, a proposal for a Robert Wood Johnson program in perinatal and infant care and development, presented to the Foundation's Policy Committee on April 27, 1973.
2. Ibid.
3. The Robert Wood Johnson Foundation. *Regionalized Perinatal Services*, Special Report Number 2, 1978.
4. M. C. McCormick and D. K. Richardson. "Access to Neonatal Intensive Care." *The Future of Children*, 1995, 5(1), 162–175; M. C. McCormick, S. Shapiro, and B. H. Starfield. "The Regionalization of Perinatal Services: Summary of the Evaluation of a National Demonstration Program," *Journal of the American Medical Association*, 1985, 253(6), 799–804.

5. K. G. Johnson. *Regionalized Perinatal Program*. Program director's report to The Robert Wood Johnson Foundation, 1982.

6. K. G. Johnson. *Report on the Foundation's Regionalized Perinatal Program*. Presented to The Robert Wood Johnson Foundation, October, 1980.

7. M. C. McCormick, S. Shapiro, and B. H. Starfield. "The Regionalization of Perinatal Services: Summary of the Evaluation of a National Demonstration Program." *Journal of the American Medical Association*, 1985, *253*(6), 799–804.

8. Ibid.

9. M. C. McCormick et al. "The Infant Health and Development Program: Interim Summary." *Journal of Developmental and Behavioral Pediatrics*, 1998, *19*(5), 359–370.

10. M. C. McCormick et al. "The Health and Developmental Status of Very Low-Birth-Weight Children at School Age." *The Journal of the American Medical Association*, 1992, *267*(16), 2204–2208.

11. The Robert Wood Johnson Foundation. *The Perinatal Program: What Has Been Learned*. Special Report Number Three, 1985.

12. R. J. Haggerty and B. Guyer. *Evaluation of Grant Made 1972 to 1992 in Maternal and Child Health*. The Robert Wood Johnson Foundation Internal Report, November, 1992.

13. J. D. Horbar and J. F. Lucey, "Evaluation of Neonatal Intensive Care Technologies." *The Future of Children*, 1995, *5*(1), 139–161.

14. S. L. Gortmache et al. "Reducing Infant Mortality in Rural America: Evaluation of the Rural Infant Care Program." *Health Services Research*, 1987, *22*(1), 91–116.

15. The Robert Wood Johnson Foundation. *Regionalized Perinatal Services*. Special Report Number 2, 1978.

16. J. D. Yeast et al. "Changing Patterns in Regionalization of Perinatal Care and the Impact on Neonatal Mortality." *American Journal of Obstetrics and Gynecology*, 1998, *178*(1, Part 1), 131–135.

17. R. M. Schwartz and R. Kellogg, *Specialty Newborn Care: Trends and Issues*. Providence, R.I.: National Perinatal Information Center, January, 2000.

18. Ibid.

19. J. D. Yeast et al. "Changing Patterns in Regionalization of Perinatal Care and the Impact on Neonatal Mortality." *American Journal of Obstetrics and Gynecology*, 1998, *178*(1, Part 1), 131–135.

20. M. K. Meynard et al. "Neonatal Mortality for Very Low Birth Weight Deliveries in South Carolina by Level of Hospital Perinatal Service." *American Journal of Obstetrics and Gynecology*, 1998, *179*(2), 374–381.

21. C. S. Phibbs et al. "The Effects of Patient Volume and Level of Care at the Hospital of Birth on Neonatal Mortality." *Journal of the American Medical Association*, 1996, *276*(13), 1054–1059.

22. M. C. McCormick and D. K. Richardson. "Access to Neonatal Intensive Care." *The Future of Children*, 1995, *5*(1), 162–175.

23. "Healthier Mothers and Babies: Trends in reducing infant and maternal mortality in the U.S.," *Morbidity and Mortality Weekly Report*, October 1, 1999, *48*(38), 849–858.

24. J.-A. Grinblat, population division at the United Nations, personal communication; estimate based on averages predicted for 1995 to 2000.

25. M. F. MacDorman et al. "Infant Mortality Statistics from the 1997 Period Linked Birth/Infant Death Data Set." *National Vital Statistics Report*, 1999, *47*(23).

26. K. D. Peters et al. "Deaths: Final Data for 1996." *National Vital Statistics Report*, 1998, *47*(9).

27. N. S. Paneth, "The Problem of Low Birth Weight." *The Future of Children*, 1995, *5*(1), 19–34; J. L. Liely et al. "Low Birth Weight and Intrauterine Growth Retardation." In L. S. Wilcox and J. S. Marks (eds.), *Data to Action: CDC's Public Health Surveillance for Women, Infants, and Children*. Atlanta: Centers for Disease Control and Prevention, 1993, pp. 185–202.

28. S. J. Ventura et al. "Births: Final Data for 1997." *National Vital Statistics Report*, 1999, *47*(18).

29. Ibid.

30. Ibid.

31. N. S. Paneth, "The Problem of Low Birth Weight." *The Future of Children*, 1995, *5*(1), 19–34. Low birthweight and very low birthweight can mean a host of problems throughout life. These babies are at risk for neurodevelopmental and other problems such as asthma, attention deficit disorder and learning disabilities. Brain injury, including cerebral palsy, occurs in 6 to 8 percent of infants weighing between 1,500 and 2,500 grams and in 20 percent of infants weighing between 500 and 1,500 grams. Although educational and social intervention can ameliorate some of the developmental problems associated with low birthweight, such programs are often expensive and are not widely available.

32. M. F. MacDorman et al. "Infant Mortality Statistics from the 1997 Period Linked Birth/Infant Death Data Set." *National Vital Statistics Report*, 1999, *47*(23); K. D. Peters et al. "Deaths: Final Data for 1996." *National Vital Statistics Report*, 1998, *47*(9).

CHAPTER NINE

⸻ Improving Dental Care

Paul Brodeur

Editors' Introduction

One aim of the *Anthology* series is to provide a retrospective look at the Foundation's work in fields where it made a contribution years ago but that are not among
its current priorities. In last year's *Anthology*, for example, Digby Diehl chronicled
the Foundation's role in establishing emergency medical services during the
1970s and 1980s. In the 1998–1999 *Anthology*, Terrance Keenan explored the
Foundation's early support, also during the 1970s and 1980s, of the emerging
professions of nurse-practitioners and physician assistants. Dentistry is another
field where the Foundation played a role two and three decades ago but has not
remained involved.

At present, the Foundation has just four grants relating to dental care out of
a total of more than 2,200 active grants. However, between 1972 and 1991 the
Foundation supported seven national programs—and many smaller ones—in the
field of dentistry. This chapter explores the variety of approaches taken to improve
the delivery and the quality of dental care. These range from scholarships for medical students to large-scale research studies and from programs to increase disabled
persons' access to dental services to developing leaders in the field.

This chapter, by Paul Brodeur, a former staff writer at *The New Yorker* who has written previously for the *Anthology*, follows the chronology of the Foundation's work in the field of dentistry. The chronology includes the following: (1) early scholarship and loan programs for dental students; (2) a program to train dentists in how to treat handicapped patients; (3) a major research study testing different ways of delivering fluoride to school children; (4) an initiative to assist hospitals in offering outpatient dental care; (5) a fellowship program to enable young dental school faculty members to study the health care system; and (6) a research program to find ways of predicting which children are at risk of developing cavities.

What emerges is a case example of the strategies the Foundation uses and the way in which they evolve to meet a changing environment. The chapter raises questions about which health concerns the Foundation should address and how long its commitment should last. In the 1970s and 1980s, when the Foundation was supporting the field of dentistry, tooth decay among poor people and lack of access to dental care was a public health problem. It remains so today; the Surgeon General stated in a report issued in May, 2000, that little-noticed disparities in dental care amount to a "silent epidemic of oral diseases" among the nation's most vulnerable citizens. Given the scope and importance of the problem, the Foundation is considering re-entering the field and funding new programs to improve oral health.

During the First World War, a Colorado dentist named Frederick McKay observed that children in certain communities exhibited severe stains on the enamel of their teeth, and in some cases disfigurement of the enamel. In dental circles, this condition became known as Colorado Brown Stain. Studies were made to determine its cause, but nothing conclusive was found until the early 1930s, when a chemist named H. V. Churchill developed a tool capable of measuring trace levels of fluorides and other salts in drinking water supplies. At that point, H. Trendley Dean, a dentist working for the National Institutes of Health, began to study the dental health status of children and adults living in more than a dozen communities with differing levels of fluorides. By the end of the decade, he was able to demonstrate that drinking water containing fluoride concentrations of up to one part per million dramatically reduced the incidence of dental caries in the teeth of children, while fluoride concentrations greater than one part per million caused brown staining and pitting that could eventually lead to the disfigurement of tooth enamel.

During the late 1930s and the early 1940s Dean published his findings in reports issued by the Public Health Service.[1] Subsequently, controlled experiments comparing the incidence of dental decay in children living in communities having fluoridated water with that of children living in nonfluoridated communities showed that the addition of fluoride to public drinking water supplies could reduce dental caries in children by more than 50 percent. It was the single greatest discovery in the history of dental medicine, and the resulting fluoridation of drinking water supplies in many communities in the nation (starting with Grand Rapids, Michigan, in 1945) is estimated to have saved hundreds of millions of dollars a year in dental restorations.

During the 1950s, Dean's discovery spawned considerable research on the use of fluoride tablets, fluoride mouth rinses, and fluoride-containing toothpaste, in order to further reduce dental caries in children. Subsequently, a number of publicly administered preventive dental initiatives—among them an extensive school-based fluoride mouth rinse program—were instituted by many communities in the nation. By the early 1970s, it was widely assumed that a combination of systemic fluorides, topical fluorides, and sealants—resin coatings to protect fissures in the occlusal surfaces of posterior teeth—could virtually eliminate dental decay in children. At the same time, it was widely recognized that the dental health of Americans could be vastly improved if they were afforded easier access to dental services. Only 25 percent of the population was receiving an annual dental checkup, and three out of every five Americans had received no dental care in the previous five years. As a result, more than half of adults over the age of 45 had begun to lose teeth.[2]

⁓ The First Dental Health Initiatives

In the autumn of 1972, the newly created Robert Wood Johnson Foundation entered the field of dental health by sponsoring and financing a $4.1 million Dental Student Aid Program—the largest single foundation grant made until then to American dentistry. Under this program, four-year grants were provided to each of the nation's fifty-six schools of dentistry to be used for scholarships or loans to women students, students from rural backgrounds, and students from the nation's black, Mexican American, Native American, and Puerto Rican populations. The program, which was administered by the American Fund for Dental Education (now known as the American Fund for Dental Health), in Chicago, was similar in intent and design to a $10 million program of student-aid grants that the Foundation had awarded several months earlier to schools of medicine and osteopathy. David E. Rogers, the Foundation's first president, who had been dean of The Johns Hopkins University's School of Medicine, described the purpose of both programs at a press conference held on October 27, 1972, to announce the dental school grants.

"The Foundation believes that the current national effort to expand the nation's output of doctors and dentists will not sufficiently benefit people in inner city and rural areas unless a substantial percentage of new medical and dental school graduates choose to practice in those areas," Rogers declared. "There is much evidence that women students, students from rural communities, and students from minority ethnic backgrounds will elect to practice in these areas more often than students from other backgrounds. Thus, we hope that by aiding schools in increasing enrollment of these students we may help to increase the proportion of students who will eventually practice in areas now sparsely served by health professionals."

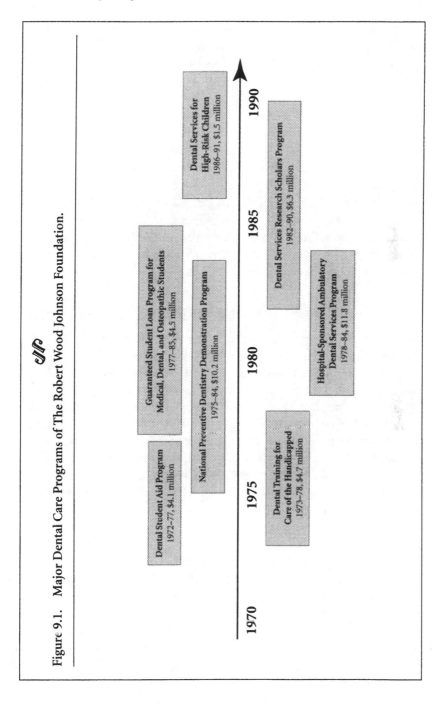

Figure 9.1.   Major Dental Care Programs of The Robert Wood Johnson Foundation.

In spite of such hopes, the Foundation's initial medical and dental student aid programs were not entirely successful, in part because targeted student aid did not prove sufficient to insure the increased enrollment of particular types of students during a period of tightened budgets and increasing costs. Undiscouraged, however, the Foundation's trustees subsequently authorized the development of a Guaranteed Student-Loan Program for Medical, Dental, and Osteopathic Students. Under this program, which ran from 1977 through 1985, the Foundation provided $4.5 million to the United Student Aid Funds, Inc., which administered the program and guaranteed the loans. In 1982, the Foundation authorized a $3 million 10-year interest-free loan to United Student Aid Funds to guarantee the existing loans. This was The Robert Wood Johnson Foundation's first program-related investment, and it was returned to the Foundation over a 10-year period ending in 1995.

⟶ Dental Training for Care of Handicapped Patients

During the early months of the Foundation's existence, Rogers and Robert Blendon, an expert in health care delivery at the Johns Hopkins Medical School, who had become vice president of the Foundation in charge of program development, sought advice on how the Foundation might best influence dental health care from John J. Salley, then dean of the University of Maryland's School of Dentistry, and from Alvin L. Morris, vice president of the University of Kentucky and president of the American Fund for Dental Education. Rogers and Blendon were enthusiastic about including dentistry in the Foundation's initial focus, and, as Salley remembers it, this enabled Morris and him "to put an oar in the water for dental programs."

One of the first proposals made by Salley and Morris was for a program aimed at increasing the number of community dentists who were trained with the appropriate skills and attitudes necessary for providing out-of-hospital dental care for handicapped children and adults. (The term "handicapped" is used in dentistry to include elderly persons and people with a variety of medical problems, as well as people who are physically and mentally handicapped.) The magnitude of the problem to be addressed was daunting. About 15 percent of the nation's then 220 million population—some 33 million people—

could be classified as physically, emotionally, or mentally handicapped. Of these 33 million people, 15 million between the ages of 25 and 65 were unable to work because they were totally disabled; 6.5 million suffered from mental retardation; 2 million were so limited in mobility that they required special help; and another 2 million were institutionalized.[3] Since many members of this large disadvantaged population were suffering from dental neglect, the essential question facing the Foundation was how to identify ways in which the dental profession could provide them with better care.

During the winter of 1973, an eight-member advisory committee established by the American Fund for Dental Education and chaired by John Salley undertook to study the problem. Salley and his colleagues soon determined that dental care for the handicapped was being provided primarily by pediatric dentists, and that most dental schools were not providing adequate instruction in how to treat handicapped people to undergraduate or predoctoral students. As a result, the limited number of trained providers of dental care for the handicapped population was imposing severe restrictions on care available in communities across the nation. Moreover, because of a lack of training and experience in dealing with handicapped people, many dentists were uncomfortable with the prospect of treating them. Others assumed that dental treatment of handicapped persons should be performed in hospitals under general anesthesia. An additional problem was the fact that, according to one federal government estimate, nearly three quarters of the nation's dental offices were physically inaccessible to the handicapped.

Operating on the premise that making permanent changes in the dental care system could best be accomplished by first making changes in the basic education of dentists, Salley and his colleagues on the advisory committee developed a pilot program designed to improve and expand the training of undergraduate dental students in providing care for ambulatory handicapped people. Such a program could serve as a long-range solution to the problem, and its designers hoped that it would demonstrate its feasibility and the practicality of the rationale behind it.

In May, 1973, The Robert Wood Johnson Foundation authorized $4.7 million to underwrite grants to eleven schools of dentistry that would introduce courses designed to train undergraduates in the dental treatment of the handicapped. The dental schools selected to receive the grants were those at Columbia University, New York University, the University of Alabama, the University of California Los Angeles, the University of Kentucky, the University of Maryland, the University of Michigan, the University of Minnesota, the University of Nebraska, the University of Tennessee, and the University of Washington. It was hoped that this cross section of institutions, representing about one-sixth of the nation's dental schools, would demonstrate whether or not dental care for the handicapped could be fully integrated into existing dental curricula, and whether or not these efforts could be sustained beyond the time when the Foundation's support would terminate.

The national program of Dental Training for Care of the Handicapped, as this pilot program was known, ran from 1973 to 1978. During that time, members of the advisory committee and other designated experts visited and monitored activities at each of the eleven schools receiving grants to make certain that the schools were complying with the Foundation's grant requirements. In the early stages, difficulties were encountered at some schools in obtaining sufficient curriculum time, in the recruitment of qualified faculty and staff, and in obtaining an adequate number of handicapped patients. In the end, however, the program to assist handicapped patients was deemed a success.

During the four years of its operation, more than 4,000 students were graduated from the full program, and 3,700 more students were taught portions of the new curricula that had been developed by the eleven schools.[4] An analysis of the program's results conducted by researchers at the Educational Testing Service, in Princeton, New Jersey, concluded that there was a clear increase in the confidence and willingness of most students enrolled in the project to treat handicapped patients.[5] Also indicative of the program's success was the decision of the American Dental Association's Council on Dental Education to include care for the handicapped as a specific teaching area to be evaluated during accreditation site visits to schools of dentistry, and the decision of the American Association of Dental Schools to develop curriculum guidelines for the care of the handicapped, and to disseminate these guidelines to all schools of dentistry.

In October, 1979, a National Conference on Dental Care for Handicapped Americans, which was designed to encourage dental schools to start programs similar to the Foundation's pilot project, was held in Washington, D.C. Supported by a grant from the Foundation, the conference was sponsored by the American Fund for Dental Health, co-sponsored by the American Dental Association and the American Association of Dental Schools, and attended by 59 representatives of dental schools across the nation, as well as by John Salley and other members of the advisory committee. (By this time Salley had become vice president for research and dean of the School of Graduate Study at Virginia Commonwealth University, in Richmond.) Chief among the topics under discussion were problems associated with implementing educational programs for teaching dental students how to treat the handicapped, such as how to obtain money necessary to set up special clinics equipped for handicapped persons, and how to find qualified faculty to teach the curricula that had been developed.

The dean of one of the schools that had participated in the Foundation's pilot program described how its continued existence had been threatened when legislative cuts in the university's budget had been passed on to the dental school. Other dental educators attending the conference also expressed concern about obtaining adequate financing for such programs. However, Salley pronounced himself optimistic that curricula for teaching young dentists how to treat handicapped people would soon be developed in all sixty of the nation's dental schools. At the same time, he deplored the lack of a clear federal legislative authority to mount a national effort to deal with the general health care of the handicapped, and warned that "the need to provide adequate dental care to 33 million handicapped Americans persists."

During the 1980s, programs for instructing dentists in how to treat handicapped patients were, as Salley had hoped, started in virtually all of the nation's dental schools, with the result that today there is no lack of dentists capable of providing care for such patients. However, the basic necessity—how to provide dental care for disabled people— still looms large more than twenty-five years after Salley and Morris identified it as being worthy of attention by The Robert Wood Johnson Foundation. Perhaps the most serious aspect of the problem is a lack of awareness on the part of state Medicaid officials of the extent of dental disease among the nation's handicapped population, and a corollary unwillingness to provide adequate fees for services to dentists who agree to treat Medicaid patients. As a result, many dentists are refusing to accept such patients. Another part of the problem is how to get handicapped people to and from the dental office, and how to make sure that they are able to keep their appointments.

Between 1986 and 1988, The Robert Wood Johnson Foundation continued its efforts in behalf of handicapped people by awarding grants to the National Foundation of Dentistry for the Handicapped, a public, nonprofit corporation, based in Denver, Colorado, that was in the process of developing a number of initiatives for dealing with dental disease among needy, elderly, and medically compromised persons. Under one of these projects, the Donated Dental Services Program, dentists were recruited to provide care free of charge to such patients. This program, which was under way in four states in 1986 when it was first supported by The Robert Wood Johnson Foundation, has now expanded into 26 states, and includes 8,000 dentists who are donating their time and effort. Program coordinators interview applicants and, if necessary, arrange for their transportation to and from dental offices.

In most cases, the costs incurred by the National Foundation of Dentistry for the Handicapped in running the Donated Dental Services Program are defrayed by grants from state legislatures. According to Larry Coffee, executive director of the National Foundation of Dentistry for the Handicapped, every dollar of state money spent on this program is returning $5.80 in pro bono dental services. Moreover, since 1986, some 26,000 patients have benefited from it. Coffee admits, however, that this and similar programs are only scratching the surface. "There are millions of handicapped people out there who need dental care," he says.

—— The School-Based Preventive Dentistry Program

Although the discovery that the addition of small amounts of fluoride to public water could sharply reduce the risk of dental decay in children was of major importance, 22 percent of the nation's population did not have access to a public water supply in the mid-1970s, and only about 50 percent of the public water supplies were either naturally or artificially fluoridated.[6] As a result, experts thought that a majority of children were developing caries. Indeed, the best available national data at the time showed that children between the ages of 6 and 11 averaged nearly one and a half decayed, missing, and filled permanent teeth, and that the rate of decay increased with age. (For example, it was estimated that adolescents between the ages of 12 and 17 averaged more than 6 decayed teeth.[7]) However, the widely held assumption that caries in children could be reduced, if not eliminated, through school-based programs using fluoride tablets, fluoride mouth rinses, fluoride-containing toothpaste, and oral health education—an assumption encouraged by the National Institute of Dental Research National Caries Program—had not been adequately tested. In fact, most studies of school-based preventive dentistry had failed to include longitudinal comparison groups—groups whose dental experience had been followed over time, in order to show whether observed changes were the result of the various preventive dentistry procedures being tested or whether the changes resulted from extraneous factors affecting the whole population.

The School-Based Program

In 1974, The Robert Wood Johnson Foundation sponsored a four-year, $2.6 million program conducted by researchers at the University of Pennsylvania School of Dental Medicine to provide restorative and preventive dental care to more than 1,800 children attending nine schools in a nonfluoridated rural county of Pennsylvania. The results were favorable in terms of reductions in untreated disease, but one of the major preventive measures—oral health education—had no measurable effect at all. In 1974, the American Fund for Dental Education approached the Foundation with the idea of conducting a national demonstration program that would determine the costs and the effectiveness of several types and combinations of school-based preventive dental procedures.

In March of the following year, the Foundation awarded a planning grant to the Fund for the development of such a program, and a separate grant to the RAND Corporation, of Santa Monica, to design data-collection procedures and conduct an independent evaluation of findings. Alvin Morris, who had become executive director of the Association of Academic Health Centers, was selected by the American Fund for Dental Education to serve as chairman of an advisory committee, and Harry M. Bohannan, a former dean of the University of Kentucky School of Dentistry, was selected as project director. The independent evaluation was conducted by Stephen Klein, a senior research scientist at the RAND Corporation, who was a specialist in research design and measurement.

Through the combined efforts of the American Fund for Dental Education and the RAND Corporation, a proposal was submitted to the Foundation for a demonstration program that would test two hypotheses: first, that a combination of fluorides and sealants would eliminate almost all dental caries in children; and, second, that the cost of school-based dental care would be low when compared to the cost of restoring tooth surfaces that would become decayed if the preventive care was not provided. In December of 1976, the Foundation awarded a grant of nearly $5 million to the American Fund for Dental Education to begin a three-year National Preventive Dentistry Demonstration Program, which was designed to determine the effectiveness of preventive dental procedures by measuring the number of tooth surfaces in children who developed caries following application of various combinations of procedures. It was also designed to determine the cost of each procedure. The program, which got under way in 1977, was later extended to include a fourth year, and by the time it ended, in June of 1983, it had cost $10.2 million, and had involved nearly 30,000 children between the ages of 5 and 14, who attended more than 200 schools in ten communities across the nation, making it the largest and most expensive dental study ever conducted.

Schools were eligible to participate in the program only if they had a high student retention rate, if they had not been involved in any previous school-based preventive dental health programs, and if teachers and school administrators had indicated a willingness to participate in the Foundation's demonstration program. To insure geographical distribution, the ten communities selected as sites were in five different regions of the nation—two each in the northeast, the southeast, the northwest, the southwest, and the central heartland. Five of the sites had optimally fluoridated water supplies, and five had been designated as nonfluoridated. Among the fluoridated communities were Chattanooga, Tennessee; El Paso, Texas; Hayward, California; Minneapolis, Minnesota; and New York City. (The study was discontinued in New York City after three years because of the high cost of running the program there.) The nonfluoridated communities included Billerica, Massachusetts; Monroe, Louisiana; Tallahassee, Florida; Wichita, Kansas; and Pierce County, in Washington State.

Enrollment in the demonstration program was open to all children who, in the fall of 1977, were in grades 1, 2, and 5 in the participating schools of each of the ten communities. (These three grades were selected because they were attended by children who were at critical ages in the development of permanent teeth.) The total population under study consisted of 20,052 children in these grades. The children received a baseline dental examination and were then enrolled in a treatment regimen that included one or a combination of preventive procedures:

- Dental sealants
- Fluoride toothpaste and gel
- Fluoride mouthwash
- Fluoride tablets
- Oral health lessons plus fluoride toothpaste and dental floss for home use[8]

All of these children received annual dental examinations for the next four years, provided they were still enrolled in the study. At the conclusion of the program, the 9,566 children who remained—children who had received both the baseline and final examination—provided a sample population that was used to measure the effectiveness of the different combinations of treatment procedures.

Children assigned to treatment regimen 6 received annual dental examinations but no preventive care, and thus served as a control group against which to compare the results of the preventive measures that had been provided to children in the other five regimens. The program had two other comparison groups: 4,320 children in grades 3, 4, 6, 7, and 8, who were examined at the beginning of the program to help predict caries levels for other grades, and 4,746 children in grades 1 through 9, who received examinations at the end of the program in order to check the decay rates that had been observed.

Some Unforeseen Results

By early 1980—the end of the demonstration program's second year—investigators comparing visual examination data with baseline data observed a startling and wholly unexpected decline in tooth decay in children of all ages who were under study. At this point, they were forced to revise their projected estimates of expected decay among these children, and to propose extending the program by one year, in part because the unexpected low rates of decay would have made evaluation of preventive efforts difficult in the three-year project originally planned. In July, 1980, The Robert Wood Johnson Foundation authorized an additional year for the program, and in December of 1981 they awarded the American Fund for Dental Health a grant to finance it.

In the same month, the National Institute of Dental Research National Caries Program released the results of a study of caries prevalence in almost 38,000 American children that had been conducted during 1979 and 1980. It showed that tooth decay in children between the ages of 5 and 17 had dropped nearly 33 percent from rates reported in Health Examination Surveys conducted in the 1960s.[9] This large decline was found in both fluoridated and nonfluoridated communities, and was thought to be the result of an increased prevalence of fluorides in the food chain, especially the use of fluoridated water in food processing and the increased use of fluoride-containing infant formulas.

As expected, the final results of the Foundation's National Preventive Dentistry Demonstration Program confirmed the general decline in childhood tooth decay levels that had been observed earlier. The study also strongly reaffirmed the value of fluoridated water in reducing dental decay. For example, children in grades 1 and 2 who lived in fluoridated communities but did not receive preventive treatment in the program experienced a 30 percent smaller increase in tooth decay than their counterparts from nonfluoridated communities. Data compiled by the demonstration program revealed that reductions in caries attributable to water fluoridation were about the same as those obtained with the application of sealants—the only school-based procedure that was found to be consistently effective in reducing decay. However, in contrast to the $23-a-year cost of maintaining a child in a sealant program, the annual per-capita cost (in 1981 dollars) of water fluoridation in five U. S. communities ranged from six cents in Denver, Colorado, to 80 cents in rural West Virginia.[10] The study also showed that the annual cost of a school-based sealant program was far more than the annual cost of restoring tooth surfaces that sealants had prevented from becoming decayed.

One of the most surprising and controversial findings of the National Preventive Dentistry Demonstration Program concerned the lack of effectiveness of fluoride mouth rinsing and fluoride tablets in preventing tooth decay in children. Guides and pamphlets issued by the National Institute of Dental Research National Caries Program had reported that the use of such procedures by schoolchildren in nonfluoridated communities could result in reductions of decay of between 20 and 50 percent, and for only $.50 to $1.00 per child per year.[11] However, according to data compiled from the demonstration program, school-based weekly fluoride mouth rinsing and daily fluoride tablets were "not consistently effective in preventing clinically significant tooth decay beyond that already prevented by typical home and dental office care."

The conclusion about mouth rinsing was particularly galling to officials of the National Institute of Dental Research, who had strongly recommended a nationwide school-based program of weekly mouth rinsing, and later tried without success to discredit the demonstration program's finding. However, Harry Bohannan, the program director, who had become professor of dental ecology at the School of Dentistry of the University of North Carolina at Chapel Hill, was unequivocal about the matter. "On the basis of our results, we can't make any strong argument that fluoride mouth rinse programs are effective enough to be recommended, considering their cost, attrition rate, and the effort required to maintain them over a long period of time," he declared. "In fluoridated communities, they are not merited at all."

In the end, Bohannan and his colleagues were able to discount the twin hypotheses that the demonstration program had been designed to test, concluding that it was not possible to eradicate tooth decay in a highly comprehensive, school-based preventive program, and that the cost of such a program for all children was prohibitive. At the same time, the data they collected during their four-year investigation led to the highly significant finding that some 20 percent of the children under study were developing fully 80 percent of the dental decay being observed. As a result, Bohannan and his colleagues recommended that the traditional approach of providing equal preventive dental services to all children be reevaluated, and that serious consideration be given to the development of a caries-prediction model that could accurately identify high-risk children and allow preventive measures to be targeted directly at them.

—— The Hospital-Based Program

Meanwhile, The Robert Wood Johnson Foundation was pursuing other initiatives to deal with problems of dental health delivery that faced the nation. Surveys taken in the early 1970s had indicated that in any given year approximately 90 percent of the population had developed periodontal disease or dental caries requiring treatment. In spite of this, only about one-third of the population was receiving comprehensive dental treatment and preventive measures necessary to avoid serious dental problems. Nearly half of the population was receiving some type of episodic care—either emergency treatment for relieving pain or for treating acute conditions—but no continual care was being provided. About 10 percent of the population, including 30 percent of all children under the age of 17, had never been evaluated or treated by a dentist. Screening programs indicated that as many as 95 percent of the children of low-income families needed dental treatment.

Several factors were thought to lie behind this widespread lack of adequate dental care. First, the general public failed to recognize untreated dental disease as a serious problem. Indeed, many people viewed dental care either as a luxury or as something to be avoided. Second, the lack of insurance coverage for dental care limited the willingness of people to seek dental treatment. And, finally, there was a serious maldistribution of dentists due primarily to the clustering of dental practices in and around relatively affluent neighborhoods.

In 1978, operating on the assumption that teaching hospitals might be able to meet the dental needs of that portion of the population which was not being adequately served, The Robert Wood Johnson Foundation launched a $11.8 million, four-year, Hospital-Sponsored Ambulatory Dental Services Program that was designed to assist hospitals in undertaking a major expansion of their existing outpatient dental care services by enlarging their existing general practice dental training programs. Under this program, which was directed by John Salley, grants of up to $500,000 each were made to 25 hospitals—most of them in inner cities or in poor suburbs—to provide 24-hour dental emergency treatment, basic dental treatment on a regular basis for patients who were without a regular source of dental care, and primary prevention and dental education, especially for children. To be eligible to participate in the grant program, a hospital was required to have a general dental care residency program, an organized dental service that provided dental treatment for inpatients and outpatients, and a twenty-four-hour facility for providing emergency outpatient medical services.

At the end of the program, the Foundation asked researchers from the School of Dentistry at the University of California, Los Angeles, and from the Graduate School of Public Health at San Diego State University to evaluate its findings, in order to answer these questions:

- Did the program improve access to dental care for previously underserved groups—in particular, the medically impaired, the poor, and the elderly?
- Was the quality of dental care provided by the hospitals comparable to that provided by private dentistry in terms of preventive care and continuing care over time?
- How did the costs of providing dental care in hospitals compare to the cost of comparable services provided by private dentists?
- What were the incentives for hospitals and third-party payers to sustain hospital-sponsored general dentistry programs?

The answers to these questions proved, for the most part, to be disappointing. The general conclusion reached by the evaluators was that the program had resulted in an increased volume of patients who were treated in the participating hospitals for dental problems, but not in an increase in the proportion of medically impaired, poor, and elderly patients who were treated. The evaluators also concluded that the program did not increase the continuity of dental care, which they defined as the transition by patients from one stage of treatment to another over time. Since continuity is regarded as the *sine qua non* of appropriate dental care, this finding was especially dismaying.

In their final report, the evaluators of the Hospital-Sponsored Ambulatory Dental Services Program pointed out, "Without prospects for increased economic viability and eventual self-sufficiency, neither public nor voluntary hospitals are likely to commit themselves to expanded dental care programs, and they are particularly unlikely to market them aggressively among the low-income and special populations that need them the most." At the same time, the evaluators warned that it was not advisable to abandon hospital-based dental care entirely, because community dentists were unlikely to be available to treat emergency dental problems among inner-city residents who were not regular patients, and because severely handicapped patients and those in very fragile health could best be treated in the hospital environment. Perhaps most important of all, they called for the expansion of third-party coverage and government funding of dental care. "One clear outcome of this evaluation is the need for such subsidization if the proportion of the nation's population who are without access to dental care is going to be meaningfully reduced," they wrote.[12]

⚊ The Dental Scholars Program

By the end of the 1970s, officials of The Robert Wood Johnson Foundation had become aware of the need to develop a group of scholar-clinicians with experience in new areas of health services research that would enable dental school faculty to better understand and deal with the changes taking place in dentistry. Among these changes were the rapid expansion of third-party coverage for dental care, an increase in large group practices, the emergence of hospital-affiliated dental programs, and shifts in the pattern of dental disease. In 1982, the Foundation launched the Dental Services Research Scholars Program, which was designed to enable talented young clinical faculty to study the financing, organization, and delivery of dental health services in the United States. Under this program, five fellows were selected annually for two-year fellowships to be undertaken at the dental schools of Harvard University and the University of California, Los Angeles. Raymond P. White, Jr., former dean of the School of Dentistry of the University of North Carolina at Chapel Hill, was selected as program director, and a national program office was established at the University's Cecil B. Sheps Center for Health Services Research.

Between 1983 and 1990, when the $6.3 million program ended, 30 scholars had completed fellowships. By the spring of 1987, the first ten scholars who had completed their studies had written 34 scientific articles that were accepted for publication in refereed scientific journals. Of greater importance was the fact that research undertaken by the scholars led to the development of many innovative policies and procedures among them clinical protocols necessary for the dental treatment of patients with AIDS. Other research drew attention to major problems of clinical decision making. Among these problems were how to determine which of the 85 percent of eighteen-year-olds who have developed wisdom teeth should have them taken out; how important is replacing a missing lower first molar with a bridge in the treatment of relatively young patients, and when and what kind of X-ray examinations should be conducted? However, in spite of general agreement that the Dental Services Research Scholars Program had proved to be of great value, officials of The Robert Wood Johnson Foundation became concerned about the future availability of outside grant funds for dental health services research, and early in 1987 decided not to finance a third round of scholar appointments.

—— High-Risk Children

One of the most important dental initiatives sponsored by The Robert Wood Johnson Foundation grew directly out of the National Preventive Dentistry Demonstration Program. When the program came to an end, in 1983, researchers who had been involved in it persuaded officials of the Foundation to finance a secondary analysis of its results, in order to determine whether there might be some important collateral findings that could be useful in developing future dental health policy. This effort was led by John Bohannan, the demonstration program's director, and by John W. Stamm, then chairman of the Department of Community Dentistry at McGill University, in Montreal, who had been a principal consultant to the program.

"The finding that twenty percent of the children were developing 80 percent of the dental decay was foremost in our minds," Stamm said recently. "Our hope was that a secondary analysis of the mass of data that had been collected so diligently by Dr. Bohannan and his colleagues would help us combine the most important risk factors in a statistical model with which we might be able to predict with a reasonable amount of clarity just who this twenty percent might be"— in other words, which children were most likely to develop caries.

The secondary analysis, which was carried out in 1983 and 1984, strongly reinforced earlier findings that children living in nonfluoridated communities were at greater risk of developing dental decay than children living in fluoridated communities. It also showed that children with deep pits and fissures in their teeth were more prone to develop caries than children with shallow grooves. In addition, it furnished evidence that a prior history of dental decay was a predictor of future caries development, and that children from poor families were more likely to be at risk of decay than children from more affluent families.

During the secondary analysis, several statistical models for predicting children who were at high risk of dental caries were developed by John Stamm, who had become a professor of dentistry at the School of Dentistry of the University of North Carolina at Chapel Hill, and his colleagues at the School of Dentistry and the University's School of Public Health. In December of 1985, The Robert Wood Johnson Foundation authorized a grant of $1.5 million to the American Fund for Dental Health for a six-year study that would further test and refine methods of identifying such children. The study, called Dental Services for High-Risk Children, was directed by Bohannan and Stamm, and it involved a series of four successive annual oral examinations of approximately 5,200 first and fifth grade children, who were equally divided between two nonfluoridated areas in the vicinity of Aiken, South Carolina, and Portland, Maine, which previous investigations had shown to be areas with high rates of dental decay and low dentist-to-population ratios. In addition to oral examinations, the study employed newly developed and relatively inexpensive screening methods to determine to what extent certain bacteria found in saliva might be predictors of dental decay. Parent questionnaires were used to collect data on the children's socioeconomic status.

When the investigation was completed, in 1991, the researchers who conducted it found that they were able to predict 65 percent of the children who would develop three caries or more over a period of four years, and 85 percent of the children who would not develop any caries at all. The investigators found that Lactobacillus—a bacteria found in saliva—was a stronger predictor of dental decay than Mutans streptococci, also found in saliva, which had previously been thought to be the chief bacterial culprit. They also determined that dental hygienists conducting visual examinations with tongue blades and mirrors could make predictions about the dental health of children that were nearly as accurate as those of dentists using dental probes. In addition, they found that first and fifth graders who came from poor and less educated families were considerably more likely to develop caries than children from more affluent and better educated backgrounds.

"One of the greatest impacts of the high-risk children study is that risk factors for dental decay have become part of the dental vocabulary, just as risk factors for various disease had previously become part of the medical vocabulary," Stamm said recently. "The question now is how to create an environment in which poor children with bad teeth can be brought to the dental chair. In my judgment, the dental public health infrastructure of the nation has fallen into disarray. It is critically important that state dental Medicaid funds be increased for less advantaged citizens, and that an educational program be established to encourage the parents of children at high risk of developing dental decay to bring them to the dentist. Equally important, parents of high-risk children must be persuaded to keep any subsequent appointments that may be made."

~~~ Conclusion

Evidence that the dental public health infrastructure of the nation has fallen into disarray is not hard to come by. Increasing numbers of dentists are refusing to treat Medicaid patients, on the ground that fees for Medicaid services are too low, and the administrators of state-run Medicaid programs are, for the most part, refusing to set aside more money for dental care. As a result, although the percentage of children who develop tooth decay has remained fairly steady over recent years, the percentage of children who get treatment for caries has dropped. Not surprisingly, tooth decay and the corollary health problems it can cause have become concentrated in the nation's poor and immigrant children, who are estimated to number between 5 and 10 million.[13]

It seems ironic that access to dental care for poor and immigrant children should still be a public health concern more than a quarter of a century after David Rogers announced The Robert Wood Johnson Foundation's first dental initiative—one designed to encourage dental students from rural communities and minority ethnic backgrounds to enter practice in inner-city and rural areas. However, John Stamm is convinced that the Foundation may still have a major role to play in the resolution of such a seemingly intractable problem. He believes that the Foundation should consider supporting a demonstration program that would educate public health officials at the state level to understand the dimensions of the growing dental crisis among the nation's poor and immigrant children, and persuade them to allocate resources from federal block grants to provide dental care for these youngsters. Such a program would also undertake to educate the parents of children who are at high risk of developing dental disease, to bring their children into the dental system.

"First, you have to make the system adequate and functional," Stamm insists. "Then you have to bring the children into it."

Alvin Morris, one of the Foundation's earliest advisers on dental affairs, suggests that the Foundation ask the scholars who were trained in its Dental Services Research Scholars Program to address the problem. "Too many kids are going to bed at night in dental pain," he says. "We need to deal with that."

Notes

1. H. T. Dean, F. A. Arnold, and E. Elvove. "Domestic Water and Dental Caries. Additional Studies of the Relation of Fluoride Domestic Waters to Dental Caries Experience in 4,425 White Children, Aged 12 to 14 Years, of 13 Cities in 4 States." *Public Health Reports,* 1942, *57,* 1115–1179.

2. M. M. Marx, "The National Preventive Dentistry Program, Foundation Rationale." Paper presented at a meeting sponsored by The Robert Wood Johnson Foundation, Scanticon, Princeton, N.J., July 28–30, 1982.

3. J. J. Salley, "Providing Dental Care to the Handicapped." *Journal of Dental Education,* 1980, *44*(3).

4. *Dental Care for Handicapped Americans.* Robert Wood Johnson Foundation, Special Report Number Two, 1979, pp. 11–12.

5. J. T. Campbell, B. F. Esser, and R. L. Flaugher, *Evaluation of a Program for Training Dentists in the Care of Handicapped Patients.* Research Report. Princeton, N.J.: Educational Testing Service, December 1982.

6. M. M. Marx, 1982.

7. *Preventing Tooth Decay: Results from a Four-Year National Study.* Robert Wood Johnson Foundation, Special Report Number Two, 1983, p. 4.

8. Schools, rather than children, were assigned to one of the six treatment regimens, because some of the procedures, such as fluoride mouth rinsing, fluoride tablets, and oral health lessons, could be administered more efficiently to classroom groups. Two of these procedures—sealants and fluoride prophy/gel treatments—were provided by teams of dental hygienists and assistants, who moved from school to school within a study community and worked under the general supervision of a dentist. The remaining preventive measures—fluoride mouth rinsing, fluoride tablets, and oral health lessons with tooth brushing and fluoride dentifrice—were administered by classroom teachers or teaching aides.

9. A. M. Miller, J. A. Brunelle, J. P. Carlos, and D. R. Scott. *The Prevalence of Dental Caries in United States Children, 1979-1980.* U.S. Department of Health and Human Services, NIH Publication No. 82-2245, Washington, D.C., Government Printing Office, 1981.

10. S. P. Klein, H. M. Bohannan, R. M. Bell, J. A. Disney, C. B. Foch, and R. C. Graves. "The Cost and Effectiveness of School-Based Preventive Dental Care." *American Journal of Public Health,* April 1985, *75*(4), p. 389.

11. J. A. Disney, H. M. Bohannan, S. P. Klein, and R. M. Bell, "A Case Study in Contesting the Conventional Wisdom: School-Based Fluoride Mouthrinse Programs in the USA." *Community Dental Oral Epidemiology, 18,* 46–56, 1990, p. 47.

12. M. H. Schoen, M. Marcus, and A. L. Koch. "An Evaluation of the Robert Wood Johnson Foundation's Hospital-Sponsored Ambulatory Dental Program." *Health Services Research* 22:3 (August 1987) pp. 327–339.
13. C. Goldberg. "Poor Children With Bad Teeth Have Trouble Finding Dentists." *The New York Times*, June 26, 1999, pp. A1, A8.

Collaboration with
Other Philanthropies

CHAPTER TEN

—∿— Partnership Among National Foundations

Between Rhetoric and Reality

Stephen L. Isaacs and John H. Rodgers

Editor's Introduction

A frequent question asked of Foundation staff members is, "How often do you collaborate with other philanthropies?" It seems that people outside philanthropy think that collaboration is a natural event, that there is a tight fraternity of philanthropies that want to work together on common problems.

In fact, as described in this chapter, collaboration among philanthropies is not so natural, and occurs less frequently than might be expected. Co-authored by Stephen Isaacs, who has written extensively on philanthropy over the past five years, and John Rodgers, a researcher at Health Policy Associates, the chapter examines partnerships involving national foundations generally and The Robert Wood Johnson Foundation specifically. It explores the theoretical and practical reasons that collaboration among foundations should make sense, why it does not happen frequently, and what elements should be in place for partnerships among national foundations to succeed. As such, the chapter should interest both policy makers and a general audience, including readers who want to understand how foundations operate.

Illustrating the discussion is a case study of a collaboration currently under way—the Turning Point Program—between The Robert Wood Johnson Foundation and the W. K. Kellogg Foundation. Turning Point seeks to strengthen the public health infrastructure in states and localities across the country. The authors take a hard look at the pitfalls and the potential payoffs associated with the partnership. They chronicle the efforts of the two foundations to attain the program's goals, but the end of the story will have to be told in a future *Anthology* chapter.

The fast growth of technology companies and the tremendous economic expansion of the 1990s increased the ranks of philanthropies in America, and the issue of collaboration will likely become more important than ever. This chapter offers a useful primer on how partnerships can work and when they are likely to be worth the great effort they involve.

J. R. K.

P
artnership among national foundations is one of those values that are preached far more than they are practiced. Like most national philanthropies, The Robert Wood Johnson Foundation does not have a strong record of collaboration. While the idea of collaboration among like-minded foundations has obvious appeal, the difficulty of forging and maintaining partnerships poses nearly insurmountable barriers and helps explain why there is so little tradition of it among national foundations. Ironically, many national foundations insist that local organizations collaborate as a condition of applying for grants, while they themselves are unable to forge such alliances on a regular basis. Understanding the dynamics behind partnerships among national foundations and examining the experience of The Robert Wood Johnson Foundation might contribute to closing the gap between rhetoric and reality.

—— Why Seek Partnerships?

There are many sound reasons that partnerships are theoretically attractive to foundations. A shared effort among foundations can signal the importance of addressing a specific problem—thereby increasing its visibility nationally and giving it a better chance of capturing the attention of the media and policy makers. Other organizations sensing the momentum may choose to lend assistance, join the collaboration, or make grants in the area. When The Robert Wood Johnson Foundation and the W.K. Kellogg Foundation decided to work together to strengthen public health systems through the Turning Point Program, their collaboration sent a message to the field that *public* health was, and should be, a priority.

Partnerships can increase the financial resources directed to addressing a problem. In the 1970s and 1980s, under the impetus of the Ford Foundation, community development corporations in inner cities grew in numbers and sophistication as a way to overcome housing shortages for the poor and to incubate economic development. Seizing an opportunity to expand the reach of these community development corporations, the Rockefeller Foundation spurred the development in 1991 of the National Community Development Initiative, or NCDI, which is cofunded by a consortium of foundations and corporations, along with the Department of Housing and Urban Development. Because the NCDI was concerned with housing, not health care, The Robert Wood Johnson Foundation initially chose not to participate; it later joined when NCDI's mission was expanded to include the delivery of health services. Working through two intermediary organizations—the Local Initiatives Support Corporation and the Enterprise Foundation—NCDI makes grants and low-interest loans to spur community development in urban areas. In three rounds of funding, NCDI has received financial commitments of $254 million.[1] When coupled with financial resources committed by over 250 local partners, this support is expected to yield $2 billion in community revitalization funding.

Partnerships can also spread the risk of funding innovative and potentially controversial new projects. Although the security of their assets coupled with the relative independence of board and staff should give foundations the courage to strike out on bold programming paths, the truth is that many foundations are timid; they do not like to have the nature of their investments criticized. Funding in AIDS and sex are good examples. In 1991, after political forces had thwarted the federal government from funding a survey on sexual behavior, justified in the context of AIDS prevention, the Robert Wood Johnson Foundation took the initial role in financing it. The effort was later joined by the Ford Foundation, the Henry J. Kaiser Family Foundation, the Rockefeller Foundation, the Andrew W. Mellon Foundation, the John D. and Catherine T. MacArthur Foundation, the New York Community Trust, and the American Foundation for AIDS Research. There is security in numbers.

Partnerships give foundations the opportunity to pool intellectual as well as financial resources by bringing different perspectives and potentially complementary areas of expertise to common concerns. Under the Local Initiative Funding Partners Program, The Robert Wood Johnson Foundation shares in the funding of projects identified by local foundations. This sharing plays to the strengths of both partners: local foundations' superior knowledge of their communities and The Robert Wood Johnson Foundation's large resource base and expertise in health. In another case, the Corporation for Supportive Housing played to the interests of three collaborators: the Ford Foundation and the Pew Charitable Trusts, which wanted to increase the number of units of housing in inner cities, and The Robert Wood Johnson Foundation, which wanted to improve health care. "Program officers from the three foundations were able to learn from one another," says former Robert Wood Johnson Foundation staff member Stephen Somers, who represented the Foundation in the partnership.

Collaboration with a more experienced foundation can bring credibility to a new foundation and help its staff learn the craft of philanthropy. Shortly after Rebecca Rimel, now the president and chief executive officer of the Pew Charitable Trusts, joined Pew, in the 1980s, she got in touch with senior executives at The Robert Wood Johnson Foundation. She wanted to gain expertise in health philanthropy from a foundation with more experience. This led to the first of several partnerships between Pew and Robert Wood Johnson—a program called Health Care for the Homeless. "These collaborations were pivotal in helping us to learn how to design programs, how to conduct evaluations, and how to use money strategically," Ms. Rimel says. "They enabled us to establish a national reach quickly." So meaningful was the collaboration that Ms. Rimel keeps a framed copy of the cover of the Call for Proposals of the Health Care for the Homeless program on the wall of her office; it is the only business-related piece of memorabilia to have such a place of honor.

Having a partner or partners can also bolster the resolve of the collaborating foundations to remain involved over the long term. One area where partnership among foundations seems to have been most effective is in creating new institutions—the Social Science Research Institute, the International Rice Research Institute, the Puerto Rico Community Foundation, the National Center for Tobacco-Free Kids, and Grantmakers in Health, to name a few, were initially supported by collaborative efforts of foundations. "It takes at least a decade for a new institution to take hold," says Susan Berresford, president and chief executive officer of the Ford Foundation. "You need to have an explicit understanding that you're going to be there in five years and ten years. Partnerships are one way of doing this, because you can all reassure one another that you're in for the long haul."

⎯ Barriers to Collaboration

Despite the potential advantages of working together, the barriers to creating and maintaining effective partnerships are so formidable that they threaten to sabotage the concept at all stages. The dearth of

collaborations among national foundations may well reflect a decision, reached unconsciously or consciously by program staffs and
boards, that they are simply not worth the effort.

In the first place, every foundation likes to see itself as fulfilling its
own distinctive and important mission. Each wants to make a difference and to fund innovative, creative solutions to social problems.
Working to fulfill somebody else's mission is often viewed as a diver-
sion of energies and resources.

In fact, the barrier is probably less one of noncomplementary mis-
sions and more one of who gets credit. Boards and staff want to have
their foundation's name on major initiatives. They want to take credit
for having developed programs—not simply being a member of a
team or, even worse, a bit player. Unlike commercial ventures, where
success is measured by rising stock prices, increased market share, and
compensation or other monetary reward, success in philanthropy is,
to a great extent, measured by public visibility and appreciation. Second billing—or even shared billing—threatens one of the reward systems that drive philanthropy.

Meshing the cultures of two or more institutions can pose a major
challenge. Foundations are on different timetables; boards require different kinds and amounts of information; the authority of program
officers varies from place to place; some foundations take a hands-off
approach with grantees, while others are very directive. Financial and
narrative reporting requirements differ among foundations. The more
foundations involved in a collaboration, the more cultures that must
blend—or at least co-exist in relative harmony. And the harder
grantees have to work to satisfy all the partners, particularly when, as
often happens, each has its own reporting requirements and schedule.

Moreover, partnerships are a hassle: time consuming, heavy on
process, and requiring an inordinate amount of time spent in meetings. For staffs and boards impatient for results, the transaction costs
are high. In the world of philanthropy, time is extremely precious; the
work involved in developing and maintaining a partnership can be
viewed as wasting a valuable asset.

Program officers receive few, if any, rewards for furthering collaborations. Foundations often judge their program staff on the basis of
the number and the quality of the grants with which they are associated; because partnerships take so long to develop and are labor-inten-
sive to maintain, they impede the work upon which career
advancement is based. Additionally, partnerships may require ceding

decision-making authority to a partner; as a result, program officers run the risk of being blamed for mistakes beyond their control.

And staff turnover can be high. Even where trust has developed, the departure of a key staff member can slow the momentum of a partnership. Each new program officer has to learn about the program and develop personal links all over again. Health of the Public, initially a collaboration between the Pew Charitable Trusts and the Rockefeller Foundation and later a partnership between Pew and Robert Wood Johnson that was designed to help academic medicine fulfill its social contract, is an example. There were so many changes in the people overseeing the program at the foundations that Jonathan Showstack, the national program codirector, observed, "The National Program Office became Health of the Public's institutional memory and source of training for the frequently revolving program staffs of the foundations involved."

With the economy booming and the stocks that form the basis of foundations' assets at all-time highs, many large national foundations have the money to fund programs themselves. Even though collaborative funding could free funds for other initiatives, many officials of the more well endowed foundations feel little financial imperative to seek out partners.

Finally, there is the danger that collaborative decision making may lead to a lowest common denominator approach and stifle innovation. Although the coalescing of many viewpoints can foster creativity, it can also lead to an exclusion of ideas outside the mainstream as decisions are hammered out on a consensus basis. Along the same lines, a partnership may give the appearance of collusion. A group of organizations may dominate thought about an issue and unduly sway the agenda of others who might have acted differently. Organizations outside the collaboration may feel that the collaborators are ganging up on their rivals.

All in all, these are powerful incentives *not* to establish partnerships and potent factors that can threaten their viability once they are established.

—— The Continuum of Partnerships

Even though every partnership is unique, on a general level, partnerships tend to fall along a continuum, as illustrated by Figure 10.1, from loose arrangements where the partners merely talk to one another to deeper collaborations where the partners cede individual control and truly merge their interests.

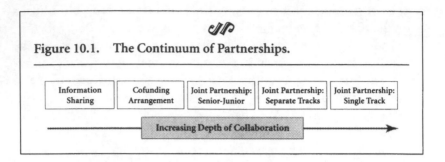

Figure 10.1.   The Continuum of Partnerships.

Information Sharing	Cofunding Arrangement	Joint Partnership: Senior-Junior	Joint Partnership: Separate Tracks	Joint Partnership: Single Track

Increasing Depth of Collaboration

Information Sharing

This is the weakest form of collaboration—if it qualifies as collaboration at all. In its most primitive form, it includes foundation presidents getting together at the Council on Foundations and other locales, program officers from different organizations talking about matters of common interest, meetings of so-called "affinity groups," and the like. Sharing information among colleagues can be a first step leading to more profound partnerships or it can be a rudimentary form of collaboration in itself—as when foundations working in the same thematic or geographic area learn what others are doing in order to avoid overlap or working at cross-purposes.

Cofunding Arrangements

Here foundations not only share information but also fund the same grantee—often buying into the vision of a strong individual able to put together a package of funding. There may be a lot of communication among the foundations, but there does not necessarily have to be. The Robert Wood Johnson Foundation has, with other foundations, supported organizations such as the National Health Policy Forum, Grantmakers in Health, and the National Center on Alcohol and Substance Abuse at Columbia University.

Joint Partnerships with Senior and Junior Partners

Sometimes a foundation has an interest in funding an activity but feels that it needs additional collaborators. In this case, the first foundation often serves as the senior partner in the collaboration. In the All Kids Count Program, for example, The Robert Wood Johnson Foundation had funds for only 15 sites in a national demonstration program to develop childhood immunization registries; by enlisting the support of the David and Lucile Packard Foundation, the Annie E. Casey Foundation, the California Wellness Foundation, the Flinn Foundation, and the Skillman Foundation, All Kids Count added nine more sites. Similarly, when The Robert Wood Johnson Foundation first considered establishing the National Center for Tobacco-Free Kids, the staff felt that the advocacy goals would be advanced and the political risks reduced if the project were undertaken in collaboration with other foundations. (The Foundation also wanted to be sure its funds were not used for lobbying purposes.) The American Cancer Society, American Heart Association, American Academy of Pediatrics, American Lung Association, American Medical Association, and the National PTA joined Robert Wood Johnson to provide initial funding to the Center.

On occasion, The Robert Wood Johnson Foundation enters a collaboration as the junior partner. In a program called Eye of the Child, The Robert Wood Johnson Foundation joined a number of other foundations, under the leadership of the Carnegie Corporation of New York, in an effort to publicize the importance of early childhood development. The Robert Wood Johnson Foundation contributed money and its staff attended periodic meetings, but it never sought to exercise leadership.

Joint Partnerships Running Along Separate Tracks

In this form of partnership, foundations fund a common grantee, but each maintains control over a specific portion of the project. Some planning may be done jointly, and meetings among the partners and grantees may be held periodically. Turning Point is an example. So is the Corporation for Supportive Housing, a joint venture among the Ford Foundation, the Pew Charitable Trusts, and The Robert Wood Johnson Foundation. Begun in 1991, this program funded affordable housing for people with AIDS and other serious disabilities. In a roughly equal partnership, the three foundations pursued their distinct but mutually supportive objectives.

Joint Partnerships Running Along a Single Track

In this kind of collaboration, a number of foundations work together to plan an initiative and then merge elements of implementation or monitoring. There might be a single national advisory committee and a single national program office. Strengthening Hospital Nursing, a collaborative effort between the Pew Charitable Trusts and The Robert Wood Johnson Foundation, is an example. Pew was interested in looking at ways to improve the health professions, and was working its way through them one at a time—dentists, pharmacists, and so forth. Robert Wood Johnson felt that it was important to prepare hospital nursing for an era of managed care. With the Health Care for the Homeless collaboration already under their belts, another collaboration involving the same parties seemed logical. Not only did the two foundations jointly fund this $27 million program, they also established a single national program office to administer it, and a single national advisory committee to provide guidance.

—— The Turning Point Program

The barriers to collaboration and the perseverance needed to navigate a partnership are amply demonstrated by the Turning Point Program, a $24-million, six-year collaboration between the W.K. Kellogg Foundation and The Robert Wood Johnson Foundation to "transform and strengthen the public health infrastructure in the United States." Like many marriages, this partnership has endured some rocky times, but both partners are still together, feel that the strengths of working in partnership outweigh the difficulties, and are determined to continue the relationship.

Turning Point, which emerged in 1996 from a web of institutional and personal relationships, began as something of a coincidence. From the early 1990s on, senior executives of the Kellogg Foundation and The Robert Wood Johnson Foundation had been meeting from time to time to explore ways in which the two foundations could collaborate. "We focused on three areas," says Tom Bruce, a former program director of Kellogg. "Public health, Native Americans, and the health professions." Parallel to these conversations, a small public health working group at The Robert Wood Johnson Foundation under the leadership of Nancy Kaufman, a vice president, and Marilyn Aguirre-Molina, a senior program officer, had been meeting to devise ways in which Robert Wood Johnson could help modernize and strengthen *state* health departments. At roughly the same time, the Kellogg Foundation, under the leadership of vice president Gloria Smith and program directors Steven Uranga-McKane and Tom Bruce, was working to develop an initiative to strengthen *local* health departments.

In November, 1996, Kaufman and Bruce attended a small meeting in San Diego of some of the key people interested in improving public health nationally. As the participants went around the table and introduced themselves, Kaufman said that The Robert Wood Johnson Foundation was looking into ways to strengthen state health departments, and Bruce said that Kellogg was thinking of doing the same thing on the local level. Kaufman and Bruce had dinner that night. "We decided that the only way to do this is together," Kaufman says. "Why have two separate initiatives when we could have a partnership?"

When the idea of a collaboration was broached at The Robert Wood Johnson Foundation, there was considerable excitement about it. After all, two major foundations working together to solve the same problem ought to have more impact than two foundations working in isolation. Bruce and some of his colleagues from Kellogg were invited to Princeton for discussions, and the principals from both foundations began to meet, share information, and make plans together.

Then the first storm clouds began to appear. While The Robert Wood Johnson Foundation was just beginning to consider how to approach the issue of improving public health, the Kellogg Foundation was pretty far down the road with *its* project. Kellogg had already decided what it wanted to do and how it was going to do it, and had made an agreement with the National Association of County and City Health Officials, or NACCHO, to manage the program. Although everybody liked the concept of collaboration, when it came down to it, the thought of bringing in The Robert Wood Johnson Foundation and involving *state* health departments was initially somewhat problematic for the Kellogg Foundation and NACCHO. "We didn't realize what we were getting into," says Vincent Lafronza, national program director of the Kellogg-funded portion of the Turning Point Program, based at NACCHO. "We had no idea that Turning Point would not move unless the states were involved." Meanwhile, some people at The Robert Wood Johnson Foundation, which was just dipping its toes into the public health waters, were developing their own reservations about the collaboration. The concerns on both sides were addressed by keeping the state and local elements of Turning Point separate for the most part. Although a single national advisory committee was appointed to provide overall guidance, two separate national program offices were designated to manage the program: NACCHO for the Kellogg-funded local health component and the University of Washington School of

Public Health and Community Medicine for the Robert Wood Johnson–funded state health component.

Cultural differences showed up almost immediately. "The two foundations have fundamentally different values," says Bobbie Berkowitz, the national program director of The Robert Wood Johnson Foundation–funded portion of Turning Point. "Kellogg is a community-oriented, grass roots kind of organization really interested in the community. Robert Wood Johnson is more large scale, systems oriented, and interested in having a major impact nationally. The differences in values and philosophy have manifested themselves throughout the life of the program—in discussions about what should be expected of grantees, how the Call for Proposals should be written, how the program should be funded, how it should be evaluated, and which sites should be selected as grantees."

The Robert Wood Johnson Foundation tends to be precise about what it expects of grantees. It prefers proposals whose success can be measured by observable outcomes. In contrast, the Kellogg Foundation tends to be less directive and more responsive to the desires expressed by the community. "Kellogg initially wanted to give local health departments very wide latitude about what they could do under Turning Point. Robert Wood Johnson had a tendency to let the health departments know what results it expected them to achieve," says Marilyn Aguirre-Molina, formerly the senior program officer at The Robert Wood Johnson Foundation overseeing Turning Point and now a professor of public health at Columbia University.

The Robert Wood Johnson Foundation traditionally develops program ideas by talking to a wide variety of people knowledgeable about a field, by digesting and refining the ideas it gathers, and, ultimately, by letting potential grantees know specifically what it wants through a Call for Proposals. Within the culture of The Robert Wood Johnson Foundation, a Call for Proposals is a detailed, carefully prepared document that is approved at the highest levels. Kellogg takes a fundamentally different approach. "We tend to send out an announcement generally describing the areas we wish to fund and ask the field for its ideas," says former Kellogg program director Tom Bruce. Steven Uranga-McKane, former lead program director for Turning Point at the Kellogg Foundation, adds, "Often, a potential grantee will simply send a letter of intent. If the idea appears to have potential, the program staff works with the grantee to shape something that can become a proposal." Merging these two approaches to announce a new program where the two foundations still weren't wholly clear about what they wanted to accomplish proved to be a challenge. As it turned out, the Call for Proposals was a compromise. It let potential grantees know in general terms about the new program to "provide support for states and local communities to improve the performance of their public health functions through strategic development and implementation processes," and informed them that certain outcomes—such as "developing and initiating a community health improvement plan to enhance policies and programs for advancing the public's health"—were expected.

At the meeting to select the sites held late in 1997, the tension between the grass roots/community-based approach of Kellogg and the national policy/systems change approach of Robert Wood Johnson quickly surfaced. Teams consisting of members of the two foundations, the two program offices, and the national advisory committee had visited potential grantees. "Kellogg has a strong commitment to communities and to diversity," says Barbara Sabol, program director at the Kellogg Foundation overseeing Turning Point. "It was very clear that the projects to be selected must reflect ethnic and class composition of the community." While committed to diversity, Robert Wood Johnson was also concerned with the potential to make policy changes that would have national significance. "Somebody from Robert Wood Johnson would say, 'We had a tremendous site visit to, say, New Hampshire or Wisconsin,'" says Susan Hassmiller, senior program officer at The Robert Wood Johnson Foundation overseeing Turning Point. "Then somebody from Kellogg would respond, 'But we need a southern rural state' or 'It's not diverse enough.'" Eventually, the two foundations agreed to fund 14 states with 41 local partners.

However, the state and local grantees were placed on different timetables from the start. Because public health was a new area for Robert Wood Johnson, the Foundation authorized only two years of funds for planning and agreed to consider additional funds for more sites and for implementation at a later time. Kellogg authorized three years of funding up front for both planning and implementation at its sites. Gloria Smith, vice president of the Kellogg Foundation, notes, "It would have been far better for both foundations to have been on the same timetable from the start and to plan the program around a common framework."

Even as these fundamental differences in values and operating styles threatened the collaboration, the partners worked together to develop the program and make it succeed. The key factors, according to former Robert Wood Johnson staff member Marilyn Aguirre-Molina, were the commitment, the good will, and the mutual trust of the key players at the two foundations and the two national program offices: "The two national program directors—Bobbie Berkowitz at the University of Washington and Vincent Lafronza at NACCHO—have been able to give the program a strong sense of stability and collaboration." Even with substantial staff turnover—within two years, the original program officials at the Kellogg and Robert Wood Johnson foundations and the original national program directors at the University of Washington and NACCHO had all moved on—the relationships among the program's leadership were, on the whole, warm, open, and productive.

Friendly relationships notwithstanding, tensions within the partnership continued. Perhaps the most important conflict arose at the time of the decline in the market value of Kellogg stock, the primary source of the Kellogg Foundation's assets, in October, 1998.[2] Shortly before the second annual meeting of state and local grantees—which, coincidentally, was scheduled to take place in October, 1998, in Phoenix, Arizona—NACCHO sent a letter to its 41 grantees informing them that because of the stock market decline, the activities of the Turning Point grantees would have to be curtailed significantly.

Neither the staff of The Robert Wood Johnson Foundation nor that of its national program office at the University of Washington knew about the letter beforehand; they were disappointed to learn about it only on the eve of the meeting. For its part, Kellogg was struggling with its own internal financial situation, which took precedence over giving advance notice to its partners. The lack of communication among the partners eroded much of the trust that had been so carefully nurtured, and had a detrimental impact on the partnership.

But the program—and the partnership—was still important to the public health community. Many people in the foundations, the national program offices, and the states and communities had worked exceedingly hard to make Turning Point a reality. Officials at both foundations felt the partnership was making a difference. "We were able to support some incredible public health partnerships that never would have occurred without Turning Point," Kellogg's

Barbara Sabol says. And there *was* a basic respect in each foundation for the strengths of the other. "The melding of the two cultures made Turning Point a terrific opportunity to learn from each other," Robert Wood Johnson's Nancy Kaufman says. "When we set up the national advisory committee, for example, Kellogg introduced us to an incredible array of community leaders whom we had not known before. The breadth and diversity was terrific." If it was possible, key staff members of both foundations felt, the relationship had to be maintained.

To put things back on track, Sue Hassmiller of Robert Wood Johnson suggested holding a retreat for the key people from the two foundations and the two national program offices. The retreat, which was held in Chicago in August 1999, turned around the flagging collaboration. Everyone recognized that the serious problems of communication and trust had to be addressed, and the participants were able to agree upon a plan of regular communication to repair the damage. The partners were then able to turn to more mundane programmatic matters, such as the whether or not to bring in additional states. The Robert Wood Johnson Foundation decided to fund seven more states.

The Chicago retreat appears to have led to a greater resolve between the foundations to communicate more fully and openly. "The next Turning Point meeting was a national Forum held in Atlanta a few months later. It was one of the best meetings I ever attended," Robert Wood Johnson's Susan Hassmiller says. "There was a complete turn-around—a sense of true collaboration. Not only between the two foundations but also among the state and local partnerships. I had this same feeling at the next Turning Point meetings as well. Things seem to be back on track."

⸺ Principles for Developing and Maintaining Partnerships Among Foundations

The experience of national foundations in developing collaborations offers a number of principles that can serve to guide future partnerships. The six principles that follow can help to identify areas where the pluses of partnerships are likely to outweigh the minuses; to structure partnerships in a way that will minimize problems; to prepare in advance for problems that are likely to occur; and to provide incentives that encourage collaborations where collaborations are appropriate.

1. *Before entering into a collaboration, each of the potential partners should conduct hard-headed analysis to be sure that the partnership will further its own priorities and that it can work with their potential partners.*

In a business partnership, such analysis would come under the rubric of "due diligence." Not only should each foundation view the partnership as advancing its own mission—which is usually pretty general—but the potential partnership should also be seen as furthering more narrow goals or objectives. "There should be clarity among all involved—board and staff—concerning a foundation's rationale for entering into a partnership and what it expects to get out of it," says Denis Prager, president of Strategic Consulting Services of Portage, Wisconsin. It is equally important that each foundation understand, to the extent it is possible, the culture and the operating style of its potential partners. Ideally, the cultures will be compatible or, at least, complementary. This means that part of the due diligence should consist of an examination of the potential partners' values, style, approach to grant making, and manner of doing business.

2. *The partners should develop clear, limited, and achievable objectives.*

Although formulating clear objectives is desirable in any case, it becomes more important when many parties—each of which can interpret things differently and is likely to undergo staff changes—are involved. Susan Berresford, president and chief executive officer of the Ford Foundation, has said that collaborations should be driven by "a clear and shared vision of what is to be accomplished."[3] William Richardson, president and CEO of the Kellogg Foundation, observed, "Clear goals prevent ambiguity and, more important, give the partnership a sense of purpose and urgency." He uses Project 3000 by 2000 as his example of clarity in goal setting. Writing in 1998, he observed, "This effort, which is funded by the Kellogg Foundation, The Robert Wood Johnson Foundation, and the Association of American Medical Colleges, has an unmistakable goal: to increase the number of African American, Native American, and Hispanic students entering the nation's 125 or so medical schools. When this partnership reaches its goal of 3,000 students by the year 2000, it will mean that 19 percent of the students entering medical schools are of minority status."[4]

3. *Build considerations of people into the planning and implement-ation process.*

It is deceptively easy to think of collaborations as arrange-ments among institutions. However, people make partnerships; institutions only lend their names. Rosabeth Moss Kanter, in a landmark study of partnerships involving 37 businesses, observes, "Successful alliances build and improve a collaborative advantage by first acknowledging and then effectively managing the human aspects of their alliances."[5]

The good will shown by the staff of The Robert Wood John-son Foundation and the Kellogg Foundation, for example, saw the Turning Point program through some rough seas. Similarly, lack of personal relationships has torpedoed a number of poten-tially fruitful partnerships. The personal element of collabora-tions can be strengthened by taking steps such as these:

- *Involve senior foundation executives—vice presidents or higher— at all stages.* The influence of a senior staff member can be important in directing attention to a collaborative program and building support for it, as well as bringing resources to bear to solve problems. Conversely, lack of support can mean that a partnership will languish. "At The Robert Wood Johnson Foundation, a partnership simply won't go anywhere without the strong support of a vice president," observes Rush Russell, a former senior program officer at the Foundation and cur-rently a consultant to it.

- *More than one or two people at a foundation should feel a sense of investment in a partnership.* Given the high staff turnover at foundations, it is unlikely that the same people who initiated a collaboration will be there at the midway point. Yet continuity and continued commitment remain important. The Health of the Public and Strengthening Hospital Nursing programs, for example, suffered because key foundation staff members left. The more people invested in a partnership, the less the poten-tial damage when staff members depart.

- *Arrange staff changes so that new staff members can overlap with departing staff members.* Since people leave unexpectedly and, sometimes, with little notice, this is not always possible. Where overlap can be arranged, programs benefit.

- *There is no substitute for face-to-face meetings, which should be scheduled regularly.* Even in an age of e-mails, faxes, and tele-conferences, the importance of meeting one's colleagues in person should not be underestimated. Jan Eldred, vice president of the California HealthCare Foundation, notes, "The Bay Area Independent Elders Program—a collaboration of three relatively big California foundations, one smaller foundation, and Kaiser Permanente—worked in large part because the CEOs of the major foundations met in person every six months or so. By the third year of the program, the presidents of all three foundations had changed and the priorities of at least one of the foundations had shifted. But because of these in-person meetings and the commitment they implied, the program continued despite the personnel and programmatic changes."

4. *Expect to face cultural differences among the partners and plan in advance how to deal with them.*

   The single most pervasive institutional obstacle to successful partnerships is differences in institutional cultures—the way the partners solicit and make grants, monitor grantees, disburse funds, provide assistance, evaluate activities, and so forth. While an organization's culture is integral to its identity and cannot be expected to change, steps can be taken to reduce and deal with the tension arising from the mingling of different cultures, among them:

   - *Recognize that cultural tensions are inevitable.* This will eliminate surprises when they occur. To the extent possible, anticipate areas where clashes are likely to occur and try to preempt them. Tom David, vice president of the California Wellness Foundation, notes, "There should be agreement on the mechanisms for decision making and group governance, a detail that is often dealt with only after a partnership has been established."

   - *Approach partnership cautiously rather than plunging in.* Co-funding arrangements, such as the 3000 by 2000 program, require less collaborative effort and ceding of authority—and, therefore, less chance of cultural clashes arising—than do more complete partnerships where planning and monitoring are done jointly. Short-term, less comprehensive collaborations can always be expanded; it is more difficult to cut back an unsuccessful partnership.

• *Keep talking.* As long as the lines of communication remain open and partners are treated with respect, overcoming differences is possible. "A partnership is like a marriage," says The Robert Wood Johnson Foundation's Susan Hassmiller. "You've got to communicate, communicate, communicate."

5. *Ensure transparency in decision making and open channels of information sharing.*

Decision making in partnerships can be a tricky business. Which decisions and issues are the prerogative of a single organization? Which necessarily involve all the organizations in the partnership? While the answer will be different in different cases, the value of openness is indisputable. Transparency involves sharing all relevant information before any decisions that may affect the partnership are made—regardless of who has jurisdiction for the decision. While transparency may not ameliorate differences of opinion or interpretation, it preserves the core ethics of fairness and shared responsibility—the pillars upon which trust is built.

6. *If partnerships are important, change the reward system to encourage them.*

Right now, program officers engaged in or trying to develop partnerships with other foundations tend to be penalized rather than rewarded. They get no credit that will advance their careers; must fight to get the program through the staffs and boards of more than one foundation; must defend against criticism of program elements included at the insistence of the partner; must attend a lot of meetings just to maintain the partnership; and, in general, must go to a lot of trouble. Program officers or senior executives seeking to advance must ask themselves the question "Why bother?" If foundations are serious about engaging in partnerships, they must find a way to reward those who attempt to create them.

—— Conclusion

Partnerships among national foundations are desirable in many, but not all, circumstances. Although they can have the decided benefits of bringing attention to a field, of increasing financial and intellectual resources devoted to a problem, and of decreasing risk in controversial fields, the pitfalls are also great. For a grantee, partnerships among funders can be a mixed blessing: on the one hand, they have the advantage of bringing additional resources, adding credibility, and lessening dependence on a single donor; on the other, they can cause a great deal of extra work and subject grantees to contradictory directions emanating from the different partners.

While every situation will have different pros and cons, there are some instances where collaborations appear more likely to be fruitful:

- Developing new institutions where every partner in a group of funders can put up money in the initial stages.
- Entering areas of potential controversy where a consortium approach can distribute risk more widely.
- Addressing large, difficult-to-solve problems like rebuilding inner cities or reducing urban poverty that require a great deal of money and lend themselves to a variety of approaches.

Before entering into a partnership, each party should be clear that the potential benefits of collaboration are substantially greater than the potential drawbacks and that the commitment of all the parties is sufficient to see the partnership through the difficult times that are likely to arise.

Notes

1. C. J. Walker and M. Weinheimer. *Community Development in the 1990s.* Washington, D.C.: The Urban Institute, 1998.
2. M. Dundjerski. "Instilling Healthy Competition." *Chronicle of Philanthropy,* December 3, 1998.
3. S. V. Berresford. "Principles for Partnership." *Ford Foundation Report,* Winter 1999.
4. W. Richardson. Speech to Grantmakers in Health on February 27, 1998.
5. R. M. Kanter. "Collaborative Advantage: The Art of Alliances." *Harvard Business Review,* 1994, *72*(4), 96–108.

~~~ The Editors

Stephen L. Isaacs, J.D., is the president of Health Policy Associates in San Francisco. A former professor of public health at Columbia University and founding director of its Development Law and Policy Program, he has written extensively for professional and popular audiences. His book *The Consumer's Legal Guide to Today's Health Care* was reviewed as "the single best guide to the health care system in print today;" his articles have been widely syndicated and have appeared in law reviews and health policy journals. He also provides technical assistance internationally on health law, civil society, and social policy. A graduate of Columbia Law School and Brown University, Mr. Isaacs served as vice president of International Planned Parenthood's Latin American division, practiced health law, and spent four years in Thailand as a program officer for the U.S. Agency for International Development.

James R. Knickman, Ph.D., is vice president for research and evaluation at The Robert Wood Johnson Foundation. He oversees a range of grants and national programs supporting research and policy analysis to better understand forces that can improve health status and the delivery of health care. In addition, he is in charge of developing formal evaluations of national programs supported by the Foundation. He has also played a leadership role in developing grant-making strategy in the area of chronic illness during his seven years at the Foundation. During the 1999–2000 academic year, he held a Regents' Lectureship at the University of California, Berkeley. Previously, Dr. Knickman was on the faculty of the Robert Wagner Graduate School of Public Service at New York University. At NYU, he was the founding director of a university wide research center focused on urban health care. His publications include research on a range of health care topics with particular emphasis on issues related to the financing and delivery of long-term care. He has served on a range of health-related advisory committees at the state and local levels and spent a year working at New York City's Office of Management and Budget. Currently, he serves on the board of trustees of Robert Wood Johnson University Hospital and chairs the board's committee overseeing construction of a new Children's Hospital in New Brunswick. He completed his undergraduate work at Fordham University and received his doctorate in public policy analysis from the University of Pennsylvania.

⟶ The Contributors

Joseph Alper is managing editor of DoubleTwist.com, an online magazine covering biotechnology, genomics, and biomedical research. During his twenty year career as a science and health care writer, he has written for a variety of publications, including *Science, The Atlantic Monthly, Harper's, The New York Times, The Washington Post,* and *Health Magazine.* During his career, he has won numerous national writing awards, including the American Chemical Society's Grady-Stack Award for career achievements in science writing and two national magazine awards from the American Psychological Association. Alper has also taught journalism and writing at the University of Wisconsin-Madison, Johns Hopkins University, the University of Minnesota, and Colorado State University. In recent years, he has also done strategic planning for the National Institute of Mental Health, the National Institute on Drug Abuse, and several biotechnology companies. He graduated from the University of Illinois at Urbana, and received master's of science degrees in both biochemistry and agricultural journalism from the University of Wisconsin at Madison.

Sharon Begley is a senior editor at *Newsweek,* where she has covered science since 1977. She has won numerous awards for her journalism, including the Clarion Award from Women in Communications, the Distinguished Achievement Award from the Educational Press Association of America, the Global Award for Media Excellence from the Population Institute, and the Wilbur Award from the National Religious Public Relations Council. She has written for *Astronomy, Family Life, National Wildlife, Redbook,* and other publications.

Paul Brodeur was a staff writer at *The New Yorker* for nearly forty years. During that time, he alerted the nation to the public health hazard posed by asbestos, to the depletion of the ozone layer by chlorofluorocarbons, and to the harmful effects of microwave radiation and

power-frequency electromagnetic fields. His work has been acknowledged with a National Magazine Award and the Journalism Award of
the American Association for the Advancement of Science. The United
Nations Environment Program has named him to its Global 500 Roll
of Honour for outstanding environmental achievements.

Allard E. Dembe, Sc.D., is associate professor in the Department of Family Medicine and Community Health at the University of Massachusetts Medical School and senior research scientist at the University of
Massachusetts Center for Health Policy and Research. Dr. Dembe is also
an adjunct professor at Harvard University, McGill University, the University of Massachusetts Lowell, and the University of Massachusetts
Amherst. He currently serves as deputy director of The Robert Wood
Johnson Foundation's Workers' Compensation Health Initiative. Dr.
Dembe's professional and scholarly interests include health policy and
health services research, occupational safety and health, social analysis
of work and health relationships, the history of medicine and public
health, and equity and social justice in health and health care. He is the
author of *Occupation and Disease: How Social Factors Affect the Con-
ception of Work-Related Disorders,* published by Yale University Press.

Digby Diehl is a writer, a literary collaborator, and a television, print,
and internet journalist. Currently the literary correspondent and
director of the MSNBC Book Club and West Coast editor of *Modern
Maturity,* his book credits include *Angel on My Shoulder,* the autobiography of singer Natalie Cole; *The Million Dollar Mermaid,* the autobiography of MGM star Esther Williams; *Tales from the Crypt,* the
history of the popular comic book, movie, and television series; and
A Spy for All Seasons, the autobiography of former CIA officer Duane
Clarridge. Previously the entertainment editor for KCBS television in
Los Angeles, he was a writer for the Emmys and for the soap opera
Santa Barbara, book editor of the *Los Angeles Herald Examiner,* edi-
tor-in-chief of the art book publisher Harry N. Abrams, Inc., and the
founding book editor of *The Los Angeles Times Book Review.* Diehl
holds an M.A. in Theatre from UCLA and a B.A. in American Studies
from Rutgers University, where he was a Henry Rutgers Scholar.

Janet Firshein is a writer who has been covering health policy and
delivery trends for 16 years. Ms. Firshein spent several years as a congressional reporter for the newsletter *Medicine & Health* and became

editor in 1990. In 1995, she began a year-long Kaiser Foundation Media fellowship to study how managed care was affecting medical education in the United States. Ms. Firshein has written for a variety of publications, including *The Lancet, Reuters Health, United Press International,* the *New Democrat,* and the *AARP Bulletin.* She also wrote a series of articles for WNET television in New York that were linked to specials on end-of-life care and drug addiction. Ms. Firshein also has done reporting for National Public Radio.

Rosemary Gibson is senior program officer at The Robert Wood Johnson Foundation. She is team leader for the Foundation's grant making to improve care for people at the end of life, with special interest in reform of health professions education, building capacity in health care systems to provide palliative care, and state and federal policy change. Her responsibilities have also included overseeing and developing new funding initiatives to improve care for persons with chronic disabling conditions and to encourage more minorities to enter the health professions. Before joining the Foundation, she served as a consultant to the Medical College of Virginia and the Joint Commission on Health Care of the Virginia state legislature. She began her professional career as a research associate at the American Enterprise Institute in Washington, D.C. Other interests include economic development and health care in developing countries. Ms. Gibson received a master's degree in public policy and finance from the London School of Economics.

Ruby P. Hearn, Ph.D., is senior vice president of The Robert Wood Johnson Foundation. As a member of the program executive group, Dr. Hearn participates in strategic program planning and serves as a special adviser to the president and as the Foundation's liaison with the nonprofit community. She has had the major responsibility for oversight and program development of initiatives in maternal, infant, and child health, AIDS, substance abuse, and minority medical education. She was a Fellow, Yale Corporation (1992–1998) and served on the Executive Committee of the Board of Directors for the 1995 Special Olympics World Summer Games in Connecticut, the Science Board for the Food and Drug Administration (FDA), and the Advisory Committee to the Director, National Institutes of Health. Dr. Hearn is currently a member of the National Academy of Sciences Committee on Science, Engineering, and Public Policy; the National

Advisory Council of the National Institute of Child Health and Human Development; the Institute of Medicine and its Board of Health Care Services; the President's Drug Free Communities Act Advisory Commission; the Council on Foreign Relations; the Goucher College Board of Trustees; and the Discovery Health Media Advisory Board. She received an undergraduate degree from Skidmore College and M.S. and Ph.D. degrees in biophysics from Yale University.

Jay S. Himmelstein, M.D., M.P.H., is assistant chancellor for health policy, director of the Center for Health Policy and Research, and professor in the Department of Family Medicine and Community Health at the University of Massachusetts Medical School. Dr. Himmelstein is national program director of The Robert Wood Johnson Foundation's Workers' Compensation Health Initiative. He previously served as a Robert Wood Johnson Foundation Health Policy Fellow for the U.S. Senate Labor and Human Resources Committee and has written numerous articles on occupational medicine and health policy.

Marguerite Y. Holloway is a freelance science writer and a contributing editor at *Scientific American.* Her work has appeared in various publications, including *Natural History, Business Week, Wired,* and *The Village Voice.* She is an adjunct professor at Columbia University's Graduate School of Journalism, where she received her master's degree and where she teaches courses on environmental and science and health reporting. She has edited and written medical and health stories for *Scientific American* since she joined the magazine's staff in 1990; before then, she covered similar topics as a reporter for the *Medical Tribune.*

Frank Karel is vice president for communications at The Robert Wood Johnson Foundation, a position he held from 1974 until early 1987 and then resumed again in 1993. During the interim years, he served in the same capacity at the Rockefeller Foundation. Mr. Karel has also served as a program officer at the Commonwealth Fund, headed The Johns Hopkins Medical Institution's public relations office, was an associate director of the federal government's National Cancer Institute, and was director of planning for National Jewish Hospital and Research Center in Denver. He began his career as *The Miami Herald*'s first science writer after having been a staff writer for *The Tampa Tribune* and the *Gainesville Daily Sun* while pursuing his undergraduate degree. He is a director of the Council on Foundations and chairs its Committee on Media and Public Affairs. He is a member and was founding chairman of the Communications Network, a member and former director of the National Association of Science Writers, a member of the Public Relations Society of America, and past chairman of that organization's Health Section. Mr. Karel received a master's degree in public administration from New York University and is a distinguished alumnus of the University of Florida College of Journalism and Communications, where he completed his undergraduate education.

J. Michael McGinnis, M.D., M.A., M.P.P., is senior vice president and director of the health group at The Robert Wood Johnson Foundation. Dr. McGinnis came to his post in 1999 from a four-year appointment as scholar-in-residence at the National Academy of Sciences. Previously, he served as Assistant Surgeon General and Deputy Assistant Secretary for Health in the United States Department of Health and Human Services, holding leadership responsibility at the federal level for disease prevention and health promotion through four administrations, 1977 to 1995. Dr. McGinnis has served as chair of various national boards and committees, including the Nutrition Policy Board, the National Coordinating Committee on Clinical Preventive Services, the Executive Committee of the Environmental Health Policy Committee, and Secretary's Task Force on Smoking and Health. He also founded the National Coordinating Committee on School Health and the National Coordinating Committee on Worksite Health Promotion. Dr. McGinnis is a fellow of the American College of Preventive Medicine and the American College of Epidemiology, and a member of the Institute of Medicine of the National Academy of Sciences. His public service recognitions include the Distinguished Service Medal, the Surgeon General's Medallion, the Arthur S. Flemming Award, the Wilbur J. Cohen Award, and the 1996 Health Leader of the Year Award. Dr. McGinnis has degrees in political science, medicine, and public policy from University of California at Berkeley (B.A.), UCLA (M.D., M.A.), and Harvard University (M.P.P.).

John H. Rodgers, M.A., is a research and editorial associate at Health Policy Associates in San Francisco. Previously, he was a research associate and statistical analyst at the Veteran's Affairs Center for Health Care Evaluation in Menlo Park, California, where he conducted national evaluation studies of substance abuse treatment programs.

His interests include social policy, international and community development, and environmental issues. He has published articles in *Medical Care*, the *American Journal of Drug and Alcohol Abuse*, the *Journal of Developing Societies*, and *Earth Island Journal*. He earned an undergraduate degree from Oberlin College and a master's degree in sociology from the University of California at Santa Barbara.

Lewis G. Sandy, M.D., is executive vice president at The Robert Wood Johnson Foundation. His responsibilities include strategic planning, program development and management, and Foundation operations. Dr. Sandy previously had been a vice president for programs at The Robert Wood Johnson Foundation (since 1991), and his portfolio of activities included grant programs for improving care for people with chronic illness; understanding the changing health care marketplace; and addressing issues of physician supply, distribution, and specialty mix. Dr. Sandy has been the Foundation's senior officer overseeing national programs to improve chronic care. He has also been active in the Foundation's workforce initiatives, in efforts to track the changing health care system, and in programs to improve managed care. An internist and former health center medical director at the Harvard Community Health Plan in Boston, Massachusetts, Dr. Sandy received his B.S. and M.D. degrees from the University of Michigan and an M.B.A. degree from Stanford University. A former Robert Wood Johnson Clinical Scholar at the University of California at San Francisco, Dr. Sandy has held clinical faculty appointments at UCSF and Harvard University and served his internship and residency at the Beth Israel Hospital in Boston. He continues to practice and teach at the University of Medicine and Dentistry of New Jersey/Robert Wood Johnson Medical School, where he is an associate clinical professor of medicine.

Steven A. Schroeder, M.D., is president and chief executive officer of The Robert Wood Johnson Foundation. A graduate of Stanford University and Harvard Medical School, Dr. Schroeder trained in internal medicine at the Harvard Medical Service of the Boston City Hospital, in epidemiology as a member of the Epidemic Intelligence Service of the Communicable Diseases Center, and in public health at the Harvard Center for Community Health and Medical Care. He served as an instructor in medicine at Harvard, assistant and associate professor of medicine and health care sciences at George Washington University, and associate professor and professor of medicine at the University of

California, San Francisco (UCSF). At both George Washington University and UCSF he was founding medical director of a university-sponsored health maintenance organization, and at UCSF he founded its Division of General Internal Medicine. Dr. Schroeder continues to practice general internal medicine on a part-time basis at The Robert Wood Johnson Medical School. He has more than two hundred publications to his credit. Dr. Schroeder has served on a number of editorial boards, including—at present—the *New England Journal of Medicine*, and is a member of the boards of the Independent Sector, the American Legacy Foundation, and the Harvard University Board of Overseers. He received honorary doctorates from Rush University, Boston University, the University of Massachusetts, and Georgetown University.

—ⁿ⁻ Index

—⁓— **Table of Contents**
To Improve Health and Health Care
1997

Foreword
Steven A. Schroeder

Introduction
Stephen L. Isaacs and James R. Knickman

Acknowledgments

Table of Contents
To Improve Health and Health Care
1998–1999

―ᴡ― Table of Contents
To Improve Health and Health Care
2000